THE HORMONE BALANCING REVOLUTION FOR WOMEN

ENHANCE YOUR DIET, FIND BALANCE, INCREASE
ENERGY, AND THRIVE; 33 DAYS TO RAPID WEIGHT
LOSS, NATURAL HEALTH REPAIR, AND HORMONAL
HARMONY

MAX HAMPTON

CONTENTS

Introduction   7

1. DAYS 1 TO 7   11
Understanding Your Hormones
Hormonal Imbalance   12
Our Body   13
Our Brain   15
Interactive Element   27
Checklist   29

2. DAYS 8 TO 12   31
Assessing Your Lifestyle
Illness   32
Age   40
Diet   44
Stress   46
Exercise   48
Medication   49
Inflammatory Triggers   50
Checklist   53

3. DAYS 13 TO 15   55
Cleaning Up Your Diet
Why Does Diet Play Such a Big Role in
Our Hormonal Balance?   56
What Is the Connection Between Our
Hormones and Our Weight Gain?   58
Rebalancing Hormones and Supporting
Weight Management   59
What Diet Is Best for Hormonal Balance
and Why?   61
What to Avoid   64

What Is Keto and Does It Help Control
Menopause Symptoms?   66
Alternative Diet Options   70
Sugar Addiction Issues   74
How to Stabilize Your Blood Sugar Levels
and Energy   74
How Can Intermittent Fasting Help
Hormones?   76
Inflammation and the Endocrine System   78
What Anti-Inflammatory Diet Is Best?   79
Women Achieving Balance Naturally   81
Interactive Element   82
Checklist   84

4. DAYS 16 TO 19   87
Mastering Your Mood
Ongoing, Unmanaged Stress   88
Why Exercise Is Key to Health and
Hormones?   91
Getting a Good Night's Sleep   97
Mindfulness Practices   102
Manage the Quality of Your Thoughts   105
How to Calm Down Fast   107
Interactive Element   109
Checklist   111

5. DAYS 20 TO 23   115
Cleaning Up Your Environment
Environmental Toxins   116
How to Reduce the Risk?   122
Checklist   139

6. DAYS 24 TO 28   141
Pills and Panaceas
The Pros and Cons of Western Medicine
and Hormone Therapy   142
Common Medications for Hormone
Imbalances   146

Interactive Element   162
Checklist   165

7. DAYS 29 TO 33   167
Making Balance a Way of Life
Homeostasis   168
Everyday Habits and Routines Affect
Your Hormones   171
How Do We Establish a New Routine?   173
How to Make Lifestyle Changes That
Stick   176
How to Get Clear of Your Lifestyle Values   179
Interactive Element   182
Checklist   183

8. REAL WOMEN SPEAK UP   185
Myths About Hormone Imbalances   186
Surviving Intense Periods During
Perimenopause   187
The Truth About Weight, Women, and
Hormones   188
Menopause Misfortune   190
Overcoming Chronic Fatigue and
Hormonal Imbalances   191
The Damage Hormones Can Do   193

Conclusion   197
References   201

INTRODUCTION

" "*Hormones get no respect. We think of them as the elusive chemicals that make us moody, but these magical little molecules do so much more.*"

— SUSANNAH CAHALAN

Elaine had always been a vibrant woman, but as she approached her thirties, she began to feel a drastic change in her body. She found herself constantly fatigued, unable to focus, and struggling to maintain a healthy weight despite her best efforts. Despite seeking medical help, Wendy couldn't find relief. She felt frustrated and hopeless. It wasn't until she discovered the power of hormonal balance that her life changed for the better.

Maria had a similar experience, struggling with chronic pain and an inability to lose weight. Despite many doctor visits and treatments, her symptoms persisted. It wasn't until she found a practitioner who understood the importance of hormonal balance that she finally saw progress and felt like herself again.

If you're reading this book, you can relate to Elaine and Maria's stories. You may struggle with hormonal imbalances and feel lost in a sea of conflicting advice and treatments. You may be tired of feeling like your body is working against you and ready to take back control of your health and happiness.

I know how you feel because I've seen the impacts up close. As a health coach, I've seen firsthand how underrepresented and misunderstood women's hormonal health can be in the traditional medical system. But after watching my long-term domestic partner suffer from endometriosis and feeling frustrated with the lack of answers from healthcare providers, I made it my mission to find a solution.

The following is what I have found. It is possible to feel good in your body. It is possible to feel at peace with your cycle, your energy level, and your fertility.

I've gathered the best available knowledge and strategies needed to balance female hormones and lessen hormonal condition symptoms. In this book, I'll share everything I've learned with you. You'll discover the shortcuts to feeling like yourself again without wasting years struggling to find solutions like Elaine and Maria.

Each chapter ends with a checklist for tracking your progress, and interactive elements throughout help to implement what you have learned. By the end of this book, you'll have the tools and knowledge needed to regain a healthy body and mind and finally feel like yourself again!

This book is the right fit for you if you're ready to take control of your health and unlock your body's full potential. So, let's get started on your journey to hormonal balance and a better life.

1

DAYS 1 TO 7

UNDERSTANDING YOUR HORMONES

> " *Hormones affect everything. Without them, there can be no life.* "
>
> — DIANA SCHWARZBEIN

I'd like you to take a moment before we get started to imagine how you'd like to feel. What would be different? What does health look like for you?

People with a menstrual cycle experience incredible hormone fluctuations as part of their bodies' natural rhythm. If even one of the hormone levels is off, the impact can feel extreme. Research shows that about 80% of women suffer from hormonal imbalances, and most of them are completely unaware of it. (Khatri, 2018). In actuality, 70% of people are clueless about diseases like PCOS that might have developed from hormonal imbalances (Teede & Boyle, 2012).

In this chapter, we'll dive deeper into hormones' role in our lives and the symptoms that are out of balance. You'll better understand what might contribute to your hormone imbalances by tracking your symptoms. We'll also explore some unexpected signs of hormonal imbalance that you may have never considered.

HORMONAL IMBALANCE

Hormones are the uncelebrated champions of our overall well-being. They regulate everything from our appetite, sleep patterns, mood, and fertility. And yet, we only pay much attention to them once something goes wrong. Maybe you've experienced some common symptoms of hormonal imbalance—like unexplained weight gain, acne, or mood swings—and wondered what was going on. Or perhaps you've never given much thought to your hormones at all.

Either way, you're not alone. A friend of mine named Alina was always tired, irritable, and prone to breakouts. She chalked it up to stress and lack of sleep, but the symptoms persisted even when she changed her lifestyle. It wasn't until she saw a doctor who diagnosed her with a hormonal imbalance that she realized what was happening.

Alina's story is just one example of how hormones can unexpectedly affect our lives. They're responsible for so much more than our reproductive health—they affect our immune system, brain function, and metabolism. When hormones are in balance, you feel full of energy, able to concentrate, and happy. But when they are unbalanced, it can cause a range of unpleasant symptoms that can be difficult to pinpoint.

If you are experiencing symptoms like these, you are ready to get started on your healing journey. This book is intended to empower you to pursue healing. With the help of your doctor, you can use this as a guide for a brighter future. So let us begin!

OUR BODY

Hormones are chemical messengers that deliver messages throughout the body. These interactions tell your organs when to start or stop a specific function. Humans produce many hormones secreted by various glands, such as the thyroid gland, adrenal gland, pituitary gland, ovaries, testes, and pancreas. Hormones act gradually, influencing multiple biological functions such as development, metabolic rate, sexual function, immunity, reproduction, and emotions. It's also important to know that each hormone has its specific function and target organ. Let's think of it this way: A post office can send thousands of letters, but each letter has a particular sender and recipient. It's the same thing with hormones. When a specific hormone enters the bloodstream, it goes to a targeted recipient to deliver the message, and an action following those instructions will come to play.

For example, one of the most important roles that hormones play in our body is regulating our metabolism. When you eat, your body breaks down the food into glucose, which is used as energy. Hormones like insulin, produced by the pancreas, help regulate the amount of glucose in your bloodstream and ensure that it gets transported to the cells that need it. If there's too much glucose in the bloodstream, the body stores it as fat for later use. If the blood has too little glucose, your body produces a hormone called glucagon, which helps release the surplus glucose stored into the bloodstream, balancing the glucose levels in the body, which will help you keep up your energy.

Other hormones like leptin and ghrelin, produced by fat cells and the stomach, regulate appetite and weight. Besides metabolism, hormones can affect every body and brain process, including mood, memory, anxiety levels, brain processes, and more. For example, cortisol, produced by the adrenal gland, is often called the "stress hormone" because it's released in response to stress and helps regulate the body's response to it. However, when cortisol levels are consistently high because of chronic stress, it can lead to adverse effects on both the body and the brain, including fatigue, depression, and anxiety.

OUR BRAIN

The endocrine system, controlled by the hypothalamus and pituitary gland in the brain, produces hormones that regulate various bodily functions. These hormones are made by glands such as the adrenal and thyroid glands and are critical in maintaining balance in the body. Hormones also have a crucial role in regulating brain function. Changes in the environment can cause chemical and structural changes in the brain, and hormones play a part in these changes. For example, thyroid hormones are necessary for the development and functionality of the brain from fetal development. It's incredible to think about how vital hormones are, yet they are often overlooked. As mentioned before, they indeed are the unsung heroes of the body.

Let's look at another way hormones affect the brain, which is through the production of the neurotransmitter serotonin. Serotonin, produced by cells in the gut and brain, helps control appetite, sleep, and mood. Various hormones, including estrogen and progesterone, can affect serotonin levels in the brain. That is why you may experience changes in mood and appetite during different stages of your menstrual cycle. Another hormone that facilitates brain function is testosterone. While often associated with male development and sexuality, testosterone is also important in the female body.

Hormones are critical in their individual roles and interact with each other to create a complex system of communication within the body. How do they interact?

Hormone Feedback Loops

Hormone feedback loops are a regulatory system that helps to maintain hormone levels within a specific range. Feedback loops regulate many hormones in which the levels of one hormone influence the production and release of another hormone.

Let's say your brain is the boss in charge of ensuring everything in your body is working correctly. One of its jobs is regulating your hormones which function as messengers that tell different body parts what to do.

The hypothalamus, a part of the brain, is a critical player in this hormone regulation game. It produces something called gonadotropin-releasing hormone (GnRH, a special signal that goes to the pituitary gland, a small gland at the base of your brain) and tells it to release two other hormones called follicle-stimulating hormone (FSH) and luteinizing hormone (LH).

These hormones then stimulate the ovaries to secrete estrogen and progesterone during the appropriate time in your cycle. As estrogen and progesterone levels rise, they provide negative feedback to the hypothalamus and pituitary gland, which helps to regulate the amount of GnRH, FSH, and LH released. This feedback loop is essential in regulating the menstrual cycle in your body.

Hormone Synergy

Hormone synergy is when two or more hormones work together to produce a greater effect than they would individually.

Let's clarify this with a short, fictional story. Imagine there was a group of superheroes who each had their special powers. One hero could create fire, another had super strength, and yet another could fly. Individually, they were each strong, but when they worked together, they were even stronger.

One day, an evil villain threatened to take over the city. The superheroes knew they had to band together to defeat him. The hero with the power to create fire used his flames to create a smokescreen to confuse the villain. The hero with super strength lifted a heavy object and threw it at the villain, while the hero who could fly came in from above to deliver a powerful punch.

Together, their powers worked in synergy to defeat the villain and save the city. Individually, they may not have been able to stop the villain, but by working together, they were able to accomplish their goal.

This same concept applies to hormones synergizing; estrogen and progesterone work together to thicken the uterine lining and prepare your body for pregnancy. During your menstrual cycle, estrogen promotes the growth of the endometrial lining in your uterus. After ovulation, progesterone takes over and helps the endometrial lining to mature, making it more receptive to a fertilized egg. Together, these hormones create a supportive environment for fertilization and implantation.

Hormone Antagonism

Hormone antagonism occurs when two or more hormones have opposing effects, and one hormone can block or reduce the actions of another hormone. For example, do you remember insulin? Glucagon and insulin have contrasting effects on blood sugar levels. Insulin promotes the uptake and storage of glucose in cells, while glucagon promotes the release of glucose into the bloodstream. Insulin prevails when blood sugar levels are high, whereas low blood glucose levels prompt glucagon secretion.

Understanding how hormones interact is essential to understanding how your body works. Hormones are complex messengers that affect many processes of your body, and their interactions are equally complex. By working together, hormones help regulate the body's functions, maintain homeostasis, and respond to changing conditions.

Forms of Hormonal Imbalance

Hormonal imbalance refers to an abnormality in the levels of one or more hormones in your body. This can occur when too much or too little of a hormone is produced, or your body cannot properly use a hormone. Hormonal imbalances can create many symptoms and health problems, depending on which hormones are affected and to what extent. Let's look at some of these imbalances.

Estrogen Dominance

As you know by now, estrogen is a sex hormone responsible for regulating your menstrual cycle, supporting bone health, and maintaining healthy skin and hair.

Estrogen dominance is a hormonal imbalance that occurs when there is an excess of estrogen in relation to other hormones in your body. Various factors can cause this, including poor diet, stress, exposure to environmental toxins, and certain medications. Symptoms of estrogen dominance may include weight gain, bloating, mood swings, irregular periods, and breast tenderness.

Low Testosterone

Low testosterone, or hypoandrogenism, is a hormonal imbalance when your body doesn't produce enough testosterone. Although this condition is often observed in men, it can also affect women. Factors leading to low testosterone include aging, specific medical conditions, and certain drugs. Symptoms of low testosterone may include reduced sex drive, weariness, despondency, and decreased muscle bulk.

Thyroid Hormone Imbalance

By now, you know that the thyroid gland produces hormones that regulate metabolism and affect almost every cell in the body, including heart rate, body temperature, and energy levels. Thyroid hormone imbalance occurs when the thyroid gland does not produce enough or produces too much thyroid hormone. Various factors can cause this, including autoimmune disorders, iodine deficiency, and certain medications. Symptoms of thyroid hormone imbalance may include weight gain or loss, fatigue, restlessness, hair loss, irregular periods, and mood swings.

Cortisol Imbalance

Cortisol is a hormone released by the adrenal gland in response to stress. It helps moderate your glucose, defense system, and blood pressure. In times of stress, cortisol levels rise to help your body cope with the stressor.

A cortisol imbalance occurs when your body produces too much or too little cortisol. Chronic stress, certain medical conditions, or medications can contribute to a cortisol imbalance. Symptoms of cortisol imbalance may include weight gain, fatigue, mood swings, and difficulty sleeping.

Insulin Imbalance

Insulin comes from the pancreas and controls your glucose levels by regulating how much sugar is in your blood. Insulin imbalance happens when the body stops responding to insulin and may result from a poor diet, insufficient exercise, or some health problems. Symptoms of insulin imbalance may include weight gain, fatigue, increased hunger and thirst, and blurred vision.

High Testosterone

High testosterone, or hyperandrogenism, is a hormonal imbalance when the body produces too much testosterone. The condition is more commonly associated with women, but men can also experience high testosterone levels. Increased testosterone may result from certain medical problems and some medicines. Symptoms of high testosterone may include acne, weight gain, hair loss, and irregular periods.

Major Symptoms of Hormonal Imbalance

Now that you have an idea of different hormonal imbalances, let's get to the part you are obviously curious about—the specific symptoms and how they occur!

Irregular Periods

Hormonal imbalances, such as estrogen dominance or progesterone deficiency, can cause irregular periods. When you have too much estrogen or do not have enough progesterone, the balance between these hormones is disrupted, leading to changes in the menstrual cycle. This imbalance can cause missed periods, longer or shorter cycles, or heavy or light bleeding. Other hormonal imbalances, like thyroid or polycystic ovary syndrome (PCOS), can also affect menstrual cycles.

Hot Flashes and Night Sweats

During menopause, estrogen levels decline, which may cause the hypothalamus to malfunction. The hypothalamus is part of your brain that helps regulate your body temperature. With low estrogen levels, your hypothalamus may interpret the body as overheated, causing symptoms such as night sweats and hot flashes.

Mood

Hormones, such as estrogen, testosterone, and progesterone, influence mood and brain function, so your mood changes if the levels of these hormones are disrupted. Low estrogen levels may induce depression and anxiety, whereas low testosterone levels can lead to irritability and mood swings.

Weight Gain

When there is an excess of insulin in your body, it can cause the body to store fat instead of burning it for energy. Insulin resistance, or type two diabetes, a condition where the body becomes resistant to the effects of insulin, is a common cause of weight gain. Other hormonal imbalances, such as insufficient thyroid hormone levels, may also trigger weight gain. Low thyroid hormone levels can slow your body's metabolism, making it more difficult to burn calories.

Skin, Nail, and Hair Problems

Low estrogen levels can cause dry skin and brittle nails, while high testosterone levels can cause acne and excess hair growth. Hair loss can be caused by thyroid dysfunction and an imbalance in the dihydrotestosterone hormone (DHT). When DHT levels are too high, it can cause your hair follicles to shrink, leading to hair loss.

Low Libido

Hormonal imbalances can affect your sexual desire and function by altering the levels of estrogen, testosterone, and other sex hormones. Low estrogen levels, for example, can cause vaginal dryness and pain during sex, while low testosterone levels can lead to decreased sexual desire and arousal in both men and women.

Insomnia or Poor Sleep

Your sleep cycle is regulated by hormones such as melatonin and cortisol. Suppose you have high cortisol levels, a hormone released in response to stress. In that case, it can interfere with melatonin production, making falling and staying asleep difficult. Another example is how estrogen can influence the production of serotonin, a neurotransmitter that helps regulate sleep. Because of this, a disruption in estrogen may also affect your sleep cycle.

Breast Tenderness

Hormonal imbalances can also cause breast tenderness or pain. Estrogen plays a crucial role in developing your breast tissue and ducts and contributes to breast tenderness. When estrogen levels rise, your breast tissue responds by retaining fluid, which can cause swelling, sensitivity, and pain. Therefore, breast tenderness commonly happens during the premenstrual phase, when estrogen levels are highest.

Headaches

Hormone changes can also result in headaches, including migraines. When you have low estrogen levels, this may cause headaches because of the hormone's effect on the blood vessels in the brain. Estrogen helps to regulate blood flow by promoting the production of nitric oxide, which relaxes blood vessels and increases blood flow. A reduction in estrogen levels can constrict blood vessels, resulting in a decline in the supply of blood and oxygen to the brain. This may trigger headaches and migraines.

Weak Bones

Low estrogen and testosterone levels can lead to weak bones and increase the risk of osteoporosis, in which bones become fragile and brittle. How? Estrogen plays a crucial role in maintaining your bone health, and low estrogen levels can cause bone loss and weaken bones. Estrogen regulates the function of osteoblasts and osteoclasts, the cells responsible for forming and breaking down bone.

Additionally, it may sustain the calcium balance. When estrogen levels decline, the activity of osteoclasts increases while the activity of osteoblasts decreases, leading to more bone breakdown than formation. Estrogen also promotes the production of collagen, a protein that gives your bones strength and flexibility. Without enough estrogen, collagen production decreases, further contributing to weakened bones.

Vaginal Dryness or Urinary Leaking

Low estrogen levels may lead to vaginal dryness, itching, or burning. Estrogen plays an essential role in maintaining the health of your vaginal tissues. Estrogen aids in keeping the vaginal lining moist and healthy while supporting the growth of beneficial bacteria. In cases where estrogen levels decrease, the vaginal tissues may dry up and become less elastic and thinner, leading to vaginal dryness. This can make sexual intercourse painful and uncomfortable and increase the risk of vaginal infections.

These symptoms are more common if you have gone through menopause but can also occur with other hormonal imbalances.

Are you ready to take control of your health and finally get to the root of your symptoms? The first step is understanding your hormones. Now, let's look at your food intake and gut health.

INTERACTIVE ELEMENT

To help you assess your hormone balance, here is a simple self-assessment checklist to rate your symptoms. You can rate yourself 1: not at all, 2: sometimes, or 3: a lot.

- Do you often feel anxious or depressed? Do these symptoms worsen during menstrual cycles, pregnancy, or menopause?

- Do you find it challenging to manage your weight, even with a nutritious diet and regular exercise?
- Has your blood pressure changed, such as becoming hypertensive or hypotensive?
- Do you usually feel fatigued despite adequate rest, hydration, and a healthy diet?
- Do you have digestive problems such as constipation, bloating, diarrhea, or nausea?
- Do you have challenges with your sleep? Do you experience night sweats or chills?
- Do you get PMS symptoms like mood swings, irregular periods, painful intercourse, or low sex drive?
- Have you experienced sudden acne breakouts or hair loss?
- Do you have a puffy, swollen, or rounded face?

If you rate 2 or 3 for more than three factors, consider seeking medical advice and getting a comprehensive hormone level evaluation

CHECKLIST

Day 1

- Complete the self-assessment above.

Day 2

- Evaluate my current lifestyle habits that may be impacting my hormones, such as sleep, diet, exercise, and stress levels.

Day 3

- Keep track of any changes I make and how they affect my symptoms, so I can continue to fine-tune my approach.

Day 4

- Make a list of any symptoms I'm experiencing and when they occur in my menstrual cycle to help identify any patterns.

Day 5

- Get hormone level testing done to understand my hormone profile better.

Day 6

- Start researching various conventional and alternative treatment options that may work for my specific hormone imbalance.

Day 7

- Make an appointment with a healthcare provider specializing in hormone health to discuss my symptoms, test results, and treatment options.

2

DAYS 8 TO 12

ASSESSING YOUR LIFESTYLE

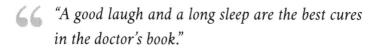 *"A good laugh and a long sleep are the best cures in the doctor's book."*

— IRISH PROVERB

Have you ever felt like something is off with your body but can't quite pinpoint what it is? It could be a hormonal imbalance, which affects many women at some point in their lives. While hormonal imbalances can have various underlying causes, evidence suggests that lifestyle factors may play a significant role. This means that simple changes in your everyday habits may positively impact your hormonal health. In this chapter, we will explore the lifestyle factors that may affect your hormones and help you identify areas that need improvement. Let's start by examining scientific evidence on what may cause hormone imbalance.

ILLNESS

Hormonal imbalances may occur for various reasons, and one of the most common causes is illness or ill health. Conditions such as polycystic ovary syndrome (PCOS), thyroid disorders, premature ovarian failure, or adrenal insufficiency can significantly impact your hormone balance. Let's look at these pathologies to help you understand them better.

Polycystic Ovary Syndrome

PCOS is a hormonal disorder that usually affects women of reproductive age and typically starts in their teenage years. It's characterized by the formation of multiple cysts on the ovaries, which may lead to an imbalance in sex hormones and disrupt the menstrual cycle. PCOS is a prevalent condition that impacts a considerable number of women of reproductive age globally, estimated to be around six to twelve percent (Mumusoglu and Yildiz, 2020).

The exact cause of PCOS is unknown, but it may be related to insulin resistance, which can cause your body to produce too much insulin. This may lead to an over-production of androgens (male hormones), disrupting your ovaries' normal functioning and leading to cyst formation.

The symptoms of PCOS can vary from person to person, but some of the most common ones include:

- Irregular or absent menstrual cycle.
- Excessive growth of hair on the face, chest, and back.
- Oily or acne-prone skin.
- Weight gain or difficulty shedding extra pounds.
- Hair loss.
- Darkening of the skin, especially around the neck, armpits, or groin (acanthosis nigricans).
- Infertility or difficulty getting pregnant.

Besides these physical symptoms, PCOS may cause the following complications:

Infertility: The hormonal imbalances in PCOS may interfere with your ovulation process, making it difficult for you to conceive.

Diabetes: As discussed earlier, PCOS is associated with insulin resistance, which may lead to high blood sugar levels and eventually type 2 diabetes.

High blood pressure: PCOS may also increase your risk of developing high blood pressure, increasing the risk of heart disease and stroke.

Metabolic syndrome: This is a common association with PCOS, and it refers to conditions such as high blood pressure, high blood sugar, abnormal cholesterol levels, and excess body fat, particularly around the waist.

Sleep apnea: PCOS puts you at a higher risk of developing sleep apnea, a condition in which breathing stops and starts during sleep.

Endometrial cancer: Having PCOS plus experiencing irregular periods or no periods at all may increase the risk of developing endometrial cancer, a cancer of the lining of the uterus.

Depression and anxiety: You may develop depression and anxiety, possibly due to the condition's impact on your body image and self-esteem.

PCOS is typically diagnosed through a combination of medical history, physical examination, and laboratory tests to assess hormone levels taken by your doctor. Treatment for PCOS may involve lifestyle changes, such as a healthy diet, regular exercise, and medications to regulate hormone levels and manage specific symptoms, such as infertility or excess hair growth.

Thyroid

Thyroid disorders are medical conditions that affect your thyroid gland, a small butterfly-shaped gland in your neck. In the previous chapter, we briefly discussed the function of these hormones, which produce hormones responsible for regulating metabolism, heart rate, body temperature, and other bodily functions. Thyroid disorders can result from an overactive thyroid (hyperthyroidism), an underactive thyroid (hypothyroidism), or an enlarged thyroid (goiter).

Hypothyroidism, or an underactive thyroid, is a common thyroid disorder that may cause you to have hormonal imbalances. Hypothyroidism happens when the thyroid gland doesn't generate sufficient thyroid hormones, which may trigger a decrease in metabolism and other bodily functions. Hashimoto's thyroiditis, radiation therapy, surgical removal of the thyroid gland, and a lack of iodine are all common causes of hypothyroidism.

The indications and symptoms of hypothyroidism may differ among individuals and may comprise: fatigue, weight gain, dry skin, constipation, depression, memory problems, and sensitivity to colds. Hypothyroidism may also cause you to experience menstrual irregularities, heavy periods, and infertility.

Hyperthyroidism is a thyroid disorder that can result in a hormonal imbalance when the thyroid gland produces excessive thyroid hormone, which increases metabolism and other body processes. Graves' disease, thyroid nodules, and inflammation of the thyroid gland are common causes of hyperthyroidism, along with autoimmune diseases.

Additionally, each individual's signs and symptoms of hyperthyroidism may differ; nonetheless, they may include; weight loss, rapid or irregular heartbeat, sweating, nervousness, and tremors. Hyperthyroidism may also cause you to have menstrual irregularities, including lighter or missed periods.

Thyroid disorders may significantly impact your hormonal health, and it's essential to consult with a healthcare provider if you are experiencing any symptoms mentioned. Treatment options for thyroid disorders may include medications, radioactive iodine therapy, or surgery, depending on the type and severity of the condition.

Adrenal Disorders

Adrenal disorders refer to medical conditions that can impact the adrenal glands, which are small organs above the kidneys. These glands produce hormones that regulate various bodily functions such as metabolism, blood pressure, and the body's response to stress. There are several types of adrenal disorders, including:

- Adrenal insufficiency: This is a condition where the adrenal glands fail to produce sufficient hormones. Other causes include infections, tumors, or the use of certain medications.
- Adrenal tumors: Tumors can form in the adrenal glands, causing overproduction of hormones such as aldosterone or cortisol.
- Cushing's syndrome: This medical condition occurs when your body produces excess cortisol, a hormone your adrenal glands generate. The primary cause of Cushing's syndrome is corticosteroid medications, but it can also result from tumors in the pituitary gland or the adrenal glands.

Adrenal disorders may affect your health in various ways, including causing hormonal imbalances. Poor functioning of the adrenal glands may cause a deficit in cortisol, leading to symptoms such as low blood pressure, fatigue, and weakness. On the other hand, Cushing's syndrome can trigger symptoms such as high blood pressure, muscle weakness, and weight gain.

Adrenal tumors may cause an overproduction of aldosterone, which can cause low potassium levels and high blood pressure.

Other additional symptoms of adrenal disorders you may experience include:

- **Menstrual cycle changes:** Adrenal disorders may cause changes in your menstrual cycle length, regularity, and intensity. This may include heavy bleeding, missed periods, or irregular cycles.
- **Hirsutism:** This term refers to excess facial and body hair growth resulting from increased androgen production.
- **Acne:** Elevated androgen levels may also lead to you developing acne.
- **Infertility:** Adrenal disorders may disrupt the delicate balance of hormones needed for ovulation and pregnancy, leading to infertility sometimes.
- **Menopause symptoms:** Having adrenal disorders may make you experience more severe symptoms of menopause, including hot flashes, mood swings, and vaginal dryness

Endometriosis

Endometriosis is a disorder in which the tissue that lines the inside of your uterus grows outside of it, such as on the ovaries, fallopian tubes, and other areas in the pelvis. This condition may cause inflammation, pain, and sometimes infertility.

The specific cause of endometriosis is still unknown, but potential explanations include the condition of retrograde menstruation, in which menstrual blood flows in the opposite direction towards the pelvis rather than out of the body, or immune system malfunctions that enable the growth of endometrial cells beyond the uterus. Other potential causes may include hormonal imbalances, genetic factors, or environmental toxins.

The symptoms of endometriosis can vary widely; you may experience mild discomfort or severe pain. Common symptoms of endometriosis may include pelvic pain, painful menstrual cramps, pain during intercourse, abnormal bleeding, and infertility. You might also feel tiredness, gastrointestinal issues, or feelings of sadness.

Endometriosis can significantly affect your quality of life and may cause infertility in severe cases. It can also lead to complications such as ovarian cysts or adhesions, which are bands of scar tissue that can cause your organs to stick together. In some rare cases, endometriosis can lead to the development of certain types of ovarian cancer.

Treatment options for endometriosis may include pain medication, hormone therapy, or surgery, depending on the severity of the symptoms and the woman's age and desire for future fertility. Early diagnosis and treatment can help to manage the symptoms and prevent further complications associated with this condition.

AGE

As a woman, it's important to understand how age can affect your hormonal balance.

Puberty

Puberty is the time in your life when your body produces more hormones, leading to the development of secondary sexual characteristics like breasts and body hair. This typically occurs between the ages of 8 and 13 but can happen earlier or later for some individuals.

The primary hormone involved in puberty for female bodies is estrogen, which handles the development of your female reproductive system and the physical changes that occur during puberty, such as the growth of breasts and pubic hair.

Perimenopause

As you approach your late 30s and early 40s, you may experience perimenopause. Perimenopausal is the transition period before menopause; your body undergoes many hormonal changes that may cause various symptoms. One of the main hormonal changes during perimenopause is decreased estrogen levels, which may lead to irregular periods and hot flashes. You may also experience mood changes, difficulty sleeping, and vaginal dryness. As your ovaries produce less estrogen, your body may have a more challenging time regulating your menstrual cycle, leading to changes in flow, duration, and frequency of periods. The drop in estrogen levels can also affect your bone health, leading to an increased risk of osteoporosis.

Other hormonal imbalances during perimenopause can include changes in progesterone, testosterone, and follicle-stimulating hormone (FSH). These changes can contribute to mood swings, acne, weight gain, and reduced libido.

It's important to note that every woman's experience with perimenopause is different, and some women may experience more severe symptoms than others. If you are experiencing symptoms affecting your daily life, it's important to talk to your healthcare provider about feasible treatment options.

The cessation of menstrual periods for 12 consecutive months marks menopause, a natural biological process that typically occurs between the ages of 45 and 55 but can also occur earlier or later. Menopause signifies the end of a woman's reproductive years. The most significant hormonal change during menopause is the decrease in estrogen levels, which can cause various symptoms, including hot flashes, night sweats, and vaginal dryness. Mood swings, fatigue, and sleep difficulties may impact daily life and well-being.

Besides the physical symptoms, menopause can also affect your bone health. Low estrogen levels can reduce bone density, enhancing the possibility of osteoporosis. Taking care of your bone health during this time is essential, such as increasing your calcium and vitamin D intake and engaging in weight-bearing exercise.

Finally, menopause can also affect your risk for certain health conditions, such as heart disease and stroke. It's essential to work with your healthcare provider to manage your risk factors and maintain your overall health during this time of transition.

Keep in mind that every woman goes through menopause differently. It's important to listen to your body and seek support from your healthcare provider as you navigate this transition.

Early Onset Menopause

Early onset menopause, also known as premature menopause, occurs when you go through menopause before the age of 40. Various factors, such as genetics, autoimmune diseases, chemotherapy or radiation therapy, surgical removal of ovaries, and smoking can cause it. Sometimes, the cause is unknown.

The symptoms of early onset menopause are like those experienced during natural menopause and can include irregular periods, hot flashes, night sweats, vaginal dryness, sleep disturbances, mood swings, decreased libido, and urinary problems. Women with early-onset menopause may also experience other health problems associated with low estrogen levels, such as osteoporosis and heart disease.

Experiencing early-onset menopause can be challenging and may affect your physical and emotional well-being. It may also affect your fertility and ability to have children. If you suspect you may be experiencing early onset menopause, it's important to speak with your healthcare provider, who can help determine the underlying cause and provide treatment and management options.

DIET

It's important to know that the food you eat can have a significant impact on your hormonal health. Your general health and wellness might be impacted by hormone imbalances brought on by an unhealthy or unbalanced diet.

Processed foods are one of the culprits that can contribute to hormonal imbalances. These foods are often high in sugar, unhealthy fats, and other additives that may contribute to inflammation and insulin resistance. This can impact hormone levels, leading to imbalances. It's important to limit your intake of processed foods and focus on a balanced, whole-food diet to help maintain healthy hormone levels.

Another food group that can contribute to hormonal imbalances is soy products, which contain phytoestrogens. Phytoestrogens are naturally occurring compounds found in plants that can imitate the actions of estrogen in the human body. While phytoestrogen may have some health benefits, consuming large amounts of soy products can contribute to imbalances in some individuals. If you're experiencing hormonal imbalances, it's best to limit your intake of soy products and focus on whole, nutrient-dense foods.

Dairy products, such as milk and cheese, may also promote hormonal imbalances in some individuals. Some dairy products contain high levels of hormones, such as estrogen and progesterone, which can disrupt the body's hormonal balance. Choosing organic dairy products can be helpful since they do not contain added hormones. Reducing your intake of dairy products or changing to organic options may be beneficial if you are battling hormonal imbalances.

Non-organic meats may also contain hormones and antibiotics that can disrupt the body's hormonal balance. These hormones can affect your hormone levels, leading to imbalances. Organic, grass-fed meats can help avoid these harmful hormones and maintain healthy hormone levels. Eating a plant-based diet or opting for plant-based protein sources can also help maintain healthy hormone levels.

Caffeine is a staple in many people's diets, but it's important to know that it can impact your hormonal health. Caffeine can increase cortisol levels, which may disrupt the body's hormonal balance. High cortisol levels can lead to imbalances in other hormones, such as estrogen and progesterone. If you struggle with hormonal imbalances, you can limit your caffeine intake or switch to alternative drinks such as herbal tea.

STRESS

As you may know, stress is an inevitable aspect of life that can be challenging to evade. However, chronic stress may cause hormonal imbalances that disrupt your overall health. By now, you have learned that when you experience stress, your body's "fight or flight" response becomes active, triggering the release of several hormones, including cortisol, adrenaline, and noradrenaline. These hormones can impact your body's hormonal balance in several ways. As previously discussed, cortisol plays a vital part in the body's reaction to stress. When cortisol levels are chronically high, it can disrupt the body's hormonal balance and contribute to imbalances in estrogen, progesterone, and testosterone.

Apart from cortisol, stress may also affect insulin levels, which can fuel insulin resistance. This can harm the body's ability to regulate blood sugar levels and contribute to insulin, estrogen, and progesterone imbalances. When insulin levels are imbalanced, it can also lead to weight gain, further exacerbating hormonal imbalances.

Chronic stress can also impact thyroid function, leading to imbalances in thyroid hormones, which can affect the body's overall hormonal balance. We have already discussed the role of the thyroid gland hormones, which include the regulation of metabolism, body temperature, and energy levels. Disruptions to this balance can lead to fatigue, weight changes, and other symptoms.

Stress can also disturb the production and regulation of reproductive hormones, such as estrogen, progesterone, and testosterone, contributing to menstrual irregularities, infertility, and other hormonal imbalances. When you experience stress, it can also interfere with your menstrual cycle by disrupting the communication between the brain and the ovaries, which can lead to irregular periods or even missed periods. It's essential to recognize the impact of stress on your body's hormonal balance and take steps to manage stress levels through relaxation techniques, exercise, and other self-care practices.

EXERCISE

Regular physical activity is vital for maintaining overall health and can positively affect hormone levels. When you exercise, your body releases endorphins, which can help reduce stress and promote feelings of well-being. However, too much or very intense exercise can also impact hormone levels and contribute to hormonal imbalances. For example, excessive exercise can lead to high cortisol levels, which can contribute to imbalances in other hormones like estrogen and progesterone.

A sedentary lifestyle can also have adverse effects on hormone levels. A lack of physical activity can lead to weight gain and insulin resistance, impacting the body's ability to regulate hormone levels. This can contribute to hormone imbalances like insulin, estrogen, and progesterone.

Adding its effects on weight and insulin resistance, lack of exercise can contribute to chronic stress. Chronic stress can lead to imbalances in cortisol and other stress hormones, impacting the body's overall hormonal balance. Therefore, incorporating regular physical activity into your lifestyle promotes healthy hormone levels.

MEDICATION

It's important to know how certain medications may impact your hormonal balance. Let's look at some types of medication and some of their known side effects.

Hormonal contraceptives, such as birth control pills, patches, and vaginal rings, contain synthetic hormones that can disrupt your body's natural hormone levels. These synthetic hormones can mimic the effects of estrogen and progesterone, potentially leading to imbalances in some women.

Hormone replacement therapy (HRT) contains synthetic hormones that may impact your body's natural hormone levels. While HRT may help alleviate symptoms of menopause, it's important to speak with your healthcare provider about this medication's potential risks and benefits.

Sometimes, selective serotonin reuptake inhibitors (SSRIs), a type of antidepressant medication, may affect hormone levels and lead to imbalances in certain people. These medications affect serotonin levels, which impact mood and other bodily functions. While they can help manage symptoms of depression and anxiety, it's essential to be aware of the potential impact on your hormonal balance.

Steroid medications, such as those used to treat autoimmune diseases and inflammatory conditions, may affect the body's natural hormone levels and contribute to imbalances in some individuals. These medications work by suppressing the immune system and reducing inflammation, but they can also impact the adrenal glands, which produce hormones such as cortisol. This may lead to imbalances in cortisol and other hormones, potentially compromising your overall hormonal balance.

Thyroid medications, such as levothyroxine, can impact thyroid hormone levels and contribute to imbalances in some individuals. These drugs are prescribed to manage thyroid conditions, including hypothyroidism. It's important to work closely with your healthcare provider to monitor your thyroid hormone levels and adjust your medication as needed to maintain a healthy hormonal balance.

INFLAMMATORY TRIGGERS

Inflammatory triggers, such as dairy, sugar, alcohol, and other foods or substances, cause inflammation in the brain or body and can significantly impact your hormonal balance. Chronic inflammation, in particular, can lead to various hormonal imbalances. For example, chronic inflammation can cause elevated levels of cortisol, a stress hormone, as you may recall, which can contribute to imbalances in estrogen, progesterone, and testosterone. This can lead to a range of issues, such as irregular periods, fertility problems, and mood swings.

Chronic inflammation can also affect the body's ability to regulate blood sugar levels, leading to insulin, estrogen, and progesterone imbalances. This can result in insulin resistance, a condition where the body is less able to respond to the effects of insulin, leading to high levels of glucose in the blood. Insulin resistance can also contribute to metabolic syndrome, leading to various health problems, including hormonal imbalances.

Chronic inflammation may also impact thyroid function, leading to imbalances in thyroid hormones. This can affect the body's overall hormonal balance, causing various symptoms such as fatigue, weight gain, and changes in the menstrual cycle.

Finally, chronic inflammation can impact the regulation of leptin, a hormone that plays a crucial role in appetite control and metabolism. When the body becomes resistant to the effects of leptin, it can result in leptin resistance, which may lead to imbalances in insulin, estrogen, and progesterone. This can lead to weight gain and metabolic problems, which can further impact the hormonal balance in women.

It's important to note that reducing inflammation in your body through diet and lifestyle changes helps you restore hormonal balance and improve overall health.

Exposure to Environmental Toxins

Exposure to environmental toxins can hurt your hormonal health. Pesticides and endocrine-disrupting chemicals (EDCs) are toxins that can disrupt your body's hormonal balance. EDCs are substances that can mimic or interfere with the function of hormones in your body, leading to hormonal imbalances. We can find these toxins in everyday products such as plastics, food packaging, and personal care products. Exposure to these harmful substances can increase the risk of developing health problems such as PCOS, endometriosis, and breast cancer.

EDCs can increase the production of estrogen. Estrogen plays a role in the development of breast cancer. Furthermore, research has shown a correlation between exposure to pesticides and a higher likelihood of developing breast cancer (Silva et al., 2019). It's important to note that the link between environmental toxins and breast cancer is complex and not fully understood. However, reducing exposure to these toxins is a precautionary measure that can help protect your health.

Taking steps to reduce your exposure to these toxins can include choosing organic foods, using natural cleaning and personal care products, and avoiding plastics and food packaging with harmful chemicals.

Remember, what you eat and how your gut processes it significantly impacts your hormone balance. Now that we have covered some root causes of hormone imbalance let's look at how our food intake affects our hormones. The next chapter will explore how making wise dietary changes promotes hormonal harmony and optimizes your health.

CHECKLIST

Day 8

- Develop a plan to manage my stress, such as practicing mindfulness or exercising regularly.

Day 9

- Assess my exposure to environmental toxins and consider making changes to avoid them.

Day 10

- Consider incorporating natural supplements or herbs into my lifestyle to support hormone balance.

Day 11

- Develop a plan to prioritize my sleep and establish a healthy sleep routine.

Day 12

- Begin a list of inflammatory triggers in my life.

3

DAYS 13 TO 15

CLEANING UP YOUR DIET

> " "Gut health is everything, it's the second brain,
> where many of our hormones are produced."
>
> — TESS DALY

This is the fun part! Eating delicious foods that nourish our bodies can be really rewarding.

Let's begin by exploring the significant impact of the food you eat and your gut health on your hormone balance. Your hormonal health is a complex and delicate system that can quickly spiral out of control because of various factors, including your diet. Optimizing your diet and focusing on foods that promote hormonal balance and gut health reduces your risk of developing hormonal imbalances and related health issues. For days 11 to 15, we delve into how your diet and gut health affects your hormones and provide practical tips on making dietary changes that can positively impact your hormonal health.

WHY DOES DIET PLAY SUCH A BIG ROLE IN OUR HORMONAL BALANCE?

Before we even answer this question, let's first understand the basic meaning of diet.

Diet refers to the foods and drinks you consume regularly in your daily routine. What you eat and drink can profoundly impact your health and well-being, affecting everything from your energy levels and mood to your risk for chronic diseases such as diabetes, heart disease, and cancer. Your food provides your body with essential nutrients such as vitamins, minerals, and macronutrients like carbohydrates, protein, and fats, which your body needs to function properly.

But how does this even connect to your hormonal balance?

Diet plays a crucial role in your hormonal balance because food provides your body with the nutrients necessary to produce and regulate hormones. By now, you already know that hormones are chemical messengers that travel throughout your body and control various physiological processes. Certain nutrients are essential for the production and regulation of hormones. These nutrients include protein, healthy fats, and vitamins and minerals like vitamin D, zinc, and magnesium. A lack of these nutrients in your diet may promote hormonal imbalances and health problems.

A diet high in processed foods, sugar, and unhealthy fats may cause inflammation, disrupting hormone production and regulation. For example, consuming excess sugar may lead to insulin resistance. When you consume too much sugar or carbohydrates, your pancreas may produce more insulin than your body needs to meet the increased demand. This may eventually result in a condition known as insulin resistance, in which the body's cells become less receptive to insulin.

When your cells become resistant to insulin, your pancreas produces even more insulin to get glucose into the cells, creating a vicious cycle of increasing insulin resistance and rising insulin levels, eventually leading to high blood sugar levels and type 2 diabetes.

Trans fats, the unhealthy fat commonly found in fried and processed foods, can adversely affect your hormone balance. Trans fats may increase inflammation and oxidative stress in the body, which can interfere with the production and activity of hormones.

Consuming a diet abundant in whole, nutrient-rich foods is crucial to sustain hormonal equilibrium and promote overall well-being. By providing your body with the necessary nutrients and supporting a healthy gut microbiome, you encourage the production and regulation of hormones and reduce the risk of hormonal imbalances and related health issues.

WHAT IS THE CONNECTION BETWEEN OUR HORMONES AND OUR WEIGHT GAIN?

Remember, hormones are crucial in moderating various bodily functions, including appetite and metabolism. When hormones become imbalanced, they can lead to weight gain, especially around the mid-abdominal section. Insulin, cortisol, and estrogen are some hormones that may impact your weight gain. We have already stressed the functions and importance of these hormones, but let's look at how they may affect your weight.

When you eat foods high in sugar or refined carbohy-drates, insulin levels can spike, causing a rapid drop in blood sugar levels and triggering hunger and cravings for more carbohydrates. This cycle can lead to overeating and weight gain over time. Elevated cortisol levels can increase appetite, cravings for high-fat and high-sugar foods, and reduced metabolism. Chronic stress and high cortisol levels may contribute to insulin resistance, leading to weight gain and difficulty losing weight.

And finally, when estrogen levels are low, the fat accumulates in the abdominal area, leading to a more apple-shaped body. This kind of fat buildup is linked to a higher likelihood of developing conditions like heart disease, type 2 diabetes, and other health issues. Now that you know the important role hormones play in weight gain, what measures can you use to balance them and manage your weight?

REBALANCING HORMONES AND SUPPORTING WEIGHT MANAGEMENT

Rebalancing hormones may be a crucial factor in achieving your weight management goals. Here are some dietary changes you can make to support hormonal balance and weight management:

- **Wholefood diets:** A wholefood diet rich in vegetables, fruits, whole grains, and lean protein sources may help regulate blood sugar levels, reduce inflammation, and support hormonal balance. Nutrient-dense whole foods can aid in the body's natural detoxification processes.

- **Intermittent fasting:** This dietary practice involves alternating periods of fasting and eating. Fasting may help regulate insulin levels and reduce inflammation, supporting hormonal balance and weight management. Done incorrectly, intermittent fasting may worsen some types of hormone imbalances so be sure to consult a doctor.

- **Cutting out dairy, sugar, and alcohol:** Consuming dairy, sugar, and alcohol in excess can contribute to inflammation and imbalances in hormones such as insulin, estrogen, and cortisol. Reducing or eliminating these foods can help support hormonal balance and weight management.

- **Healing your gut:** A healthy microbiome supports hormonal balance and weight management. Consuming probiotic-rich foods such as yogurt, kimchi, and sauerkraut can help support gut health.

- **Managing stress:** Chronic stress can lead to imbalances in cortisol, insulin, and estrogen, contributing to weight gain. Engaging in stress-management practices like yoga, meditation, or deep breathing exercises can be beneficial in promoting hormonal balance and managing weight.

- **Sleeping better:** Poor sleep habits can lead to hormone imbalances such as cortisol, leptin, and ghrelin, contributing to weight gain. Good sleep hygiene habits, such as avoiding caffeine and electronics before bedtime, can help support hormonal balance and weight management.
- **Movement:** Regular physical activity can help regulate insulin levels, reduce inflammation, and support hormonal balance and weight management.

These dietary and lifestyle changes support hormonal balance, promote weight management, and improve well-being.

WHAT DIET IS BEST FOR HORMONAL BALANCE AND WHY?

As individual hormone imbalances require different approaches, a single diet will not work for everybody. However, a diet focused on whole foods and anti-inflammatory results may benefit overall hormonal health. This diet focuses on consuming foods high in nutrients, such as fruits, vegetables, whole grains, lean protein, and healthy fats. It also involves restricting or avoiding processed foods, sugar, and alcohol. Whole foods provide your body with essential nutrients that help support hormone production, metabolism, and general function.

Foods high in omega-3 fatty acids, such as fatty fish, nuts, and seeds, may help reduce inflammation and support healthy hormone levels. Similarly, cruciferous vegetables like broccoli and cauliflower contain compounds that help the body detoxify excess hormones, such as estrogen, from the body. Foods high in fiber, such as beans and lentils, can help regulate blood sugar levels and improve insulin sensitivity, benefiting women with conditions such as PCOS.

How Can Diet Improve Your Mood?

The food you eat can have a significant impact on your mood. Certain foods can boost the production of neurotransmitters such as serotonin, dopamine, and norepinephrine, which regulate mood. Foods high in tryptophan, such as turkey, eggs, and spinach, can increase serotonin levels. Whole foods high in tyrosine, such as almonds, avocados, and bananas, can increase dopamine and norepinephrine levels.

General Good-Mood Foods

Certain foods have a positive impact on mood. Foods rich in omega-3 fatty acids are great for lowering symptoms of depression and anxiety. Foods rich in probiotics, such as kefir, yogurt, and sauerkraut, can improve gut health and positively affect mood. In addition, foods high in antioxidants, such as berries, leafy greens, and dark chocolate, can help reduce inflammation, which has been linked to depression.

Hormone-Happy Foods

Hormone-happy foods may help you balance hormones and promote overall hormonal health. These foods are rich in omega-3 fatty acids, antioxidants, fiber, and other beneficial compounds that can help regulate hormone levels.

Some examples of hormone-happy foods include:

- **Fatty fish:** Fatty fish such as salmon, tuna, and sardines are rich in omega-3 fatty acids, which help regulate hormone levels and alleviate inflammation.
- **Nuts and seeds:** Nuts and seeds are a great source of healthy fats and minerals, such as zinc and magnesium, which can support hormonal health. Almonds, flaxseeds, and walnuts are some examples of such foods.
- **Leafy greens:** Leafy greens such as spinach, kale, and cabbage are rich in vitamins and minerals, including calcium, vitamin K, and

iron, which can help support hormonal health and reduce inflammation.

- **Berries:** Berries, such as blueberries, strawberries, and raspberries, contain high amounts of antioxidants that can assist in reducing inflammation and promoting hormonal well-being.
- **Fermented foods:** Fermented foods such as yogurt, kefir, and kimchi contain beneficial probiotics that can help support gut health and improve hormonal balance.

WHAT TO AVOID

Certain foods can negatively affect hormonal balance and should be avoided or limited when supporting your hormones or overall health. Keep in mind that your body wants to heal. Eating 100% healthy can sometimes be difficult in our world. Don't worry about being perfect, just make a plan to eat as much good stuff as you can. Find every opportunity to squeeze in the hormone-healthy superfood that you can but don't stress about eating a cookie. The stress may do more damage than the cookie. Still, it's essential to know that certain foods are not fighting beside you in this battle for better health.

- **Processed foods:** Processed foods often contain high amounts of refined sugars, unhealthy fats, and chemical additives that can disrupt the endocrine system and cause hormonal imbalances.

- **Sugary foods and beverages:** Foods and drinks with high amounts of added sugars can cause a rapid spike in blood sugar levels, leading to an increase in insulin levels and contributing to insulin resistance, which may cause imbalances in other hormones like estrogen, testosterone, and progesterone.

- **Alcohol:** Excessive alcohol consumption can affect the liver's ability to metabolize estrogen, leading to a buildup of the hormone in the body. As a result, this could raise the possibility of developing breast cancer and other irregularities in hormone levels.

- **Soy products:** Soy products like soy milk and tofu contain phytoestrogens, which are plant-based compounds that can imitate the effects of estrogen in the human body. While small amounts of phytoestrogens are unlikely to cause harm, excessive intake may lead to hormonal imbalances.

- **Caffeine:** Caffeine consumption may increase cortisol levels, which can contribute to hormonal imbalances. Additionally, caffeine can interfere with the absorption of certain essential nutrients for hormone health, such as magnesium and B vitamins.

Avoiding or limiting these foods helps support your hormone health and improve your wellness.

WHAT IS KETO AND DOES IT HELP CONTROL MENOPAUSE SYMPTOMS?

Everyone has heard of the keto diet, but what exactly is it, and what does it even do for you?

The ketogenic diet, commonly known as "keto," is a low-carbohydrate, high-fat diet that aims to shift your body into ketosis. When in a state of ketosis, your body utilizes fat as an energy source rather than relying on carbohydrates. Ketosis is achieved by significantly reducing your carbohydrate intake and increasing your fat intake.

When you eat a high-carbohydrate meal, your body converts the carbs into glucose, which is the primary energy source for your cells. When you reduce your carbohydrate intake, your body doesn't have enough glucose to use for energy, so it starts breaking down stored fat instead. This process generates ketones, which can serve as an energy source for the body instead of relying on glucose.

Can the ketogenic diet be beneficial in alleviating symptoms of menopause?

During menopause, you may have fluctuations in blood sugar levels due to hormone changes. Following a keto diet may stabilize your blood sugar levels and reduce these symptoms. In addition, the keto diet might alleviate other typical symptoms of menopause, like decreased sexual desire and vaginal dryness. A keto diet may relieve inflammation, which can contribute to these symptoms.

However, it's important to note that more research is needed in this area, and the keto diet may only be suitable for some. Some women may find that a more balanced approach to nutrition, including a variety of whole foods and macronutrients, better fits their lifestyle and health goals. Speaking with a healthcare professional before making significant dietary changes is always a good idea.

What Are The Potential Benefits And Side Effects of Keto Diet?

A ketogenic diet has several advantages. It may help you lose weight, regulate blood sugar levels, decrease inflammation, boost energy levels, and enhance mental clarity.

The keto diet's main advantage is its capacity to aid in weight loss. As explained earlier, when you restrict carbohydrates, your body burns fat for fuel instead of glucose. This may result in significant weight loss, especially in the first few weeks of the diet. Additionally, the keto diet may reduce body fat, particularly in the abdominal area.

Limiting the intake of carbohydrates gives the keto diet the potential to enhance blood sugar control, leading to an improvement in insulin sensitivity and a decrease in blood sugar levels. This benefit can be beneficial for people with type 2 diabetes or those who are prone to developing insulin resistance.

The keto diet may have anti-inflammatory effects. Restricting carbohydrates reduces the production of inflammatory molecules in the body, which helps reduce inflammation. This could be advantageous if you struggle with medical conditions like arthritis, inflammatory bowel disease, or other inflammatory ailments.

Some individuals have reported experiencing higher energy levels and improved cognitive function when following a ketogenic diet. This may be because your body is using fat for fuel instead of glucose, which can result in more stable energy levels throughout the day.

Side Effects

While the keto diet may have many potential benefits, there are also some possible side effects that you should be aware of. Below are some of the most frequently experienced adverse effects of the ketogenic diet.

- **The keto flu:** Many people experience flu-like symptoms when they first start a keto diet, including fatigue, headaches, and nausea. Usually, these symptoms subside in a few days or weeks.
- **Digestive issues:** Some people experience constipation or diarrhea following a keto diet due to a lack of fiber in the diet or changes in gut bacteria.
- **Electrolyte imbalances:** When you restrict carbohydrates, your body excretes more water and electrolytes, such as sodium and potassium,

leading to electrolyte imbalances, which can cause muscle cramps, headaches, and fatigue.

- **Nutrient deficiencies:** Because the keto diet is deficient in carbohydrates, getting enough vitamins and minerals from food alone can be challenging. This can lead to nutrient deficiencies if the diet is not balanced correctly.

- **Increased risk of kidney stones:** Some research suggests that following a keto diet may increase the risk of kidney stones, particularly in people prone to the condition.

Note that these side effects may only be experienced by some who follow a ketogenic diet. You can manage or prevent these side effects by adequately balancing your diet and staying hydrated. If you're considering starting a keto diet, it's a good idea to talk to your doctor or a registered dietician to ensure the diet is appropriate for you.

ALTERNATIVE DIET OPTIONS

Aside from keto, are there any alternative diets to help balance your hormones? The answer is yes. Below are other options you may explore.

The Mediterranean Diet

The Mediterranean Diet is a healthy and balanced diet focusing on whole, unprocessed foods like fruits, vegetables, legumes, nuts, seeds, and whole grains. It also includes moderate amounts of fish, lean proteins, and healthy fats such as olive oil. The Mediterranean diet may help balance hormones, particularly insulin, and estrogen. The diet contains abundant fiber, vitamins, and minerals that aid in controlling your blood sugar and insulin levels. It also includes foods high in phytoestrogens, such as legumes and nuts, which may help balance estrogen levels. The diet's emphasis on anti-inflammatory foods and healthy fats may also help reduce inflammation and support overall hormone health.

Plant-Based Diet

This diet centers around plant-based foods as the primary source of nutrition, including fruits, vegetables, whole grains, legumes, nuts, and seeds. Plant-based diets are rich in fiber, vitamins, and minerals that help balance hormones, particularly insulin and estrogen. Plant-based diets may help improve insulin sensitivity, lower inflammation, and reduce the risk of hormone-related conditions such as breast cancer and

PCOS. Plant-based diets also have a lower glycemic load, which may help balance blood sugar and insulin levels.

Low-Carb Diet

This eating plan emphasizes protein, healthy fats, and low-carbohydrate vegetables. This diet may help you balance hormones by reducing insulin levels, which is particularly beneficial if you have insulin resistance or PCOS. Low-carb diets may also help promote weight loss, positively impacting hormone levels. In addition, low-carb diets may improve blood lipid levels, reducing the risk of heart disease and other hormone-related conditions.

It's important to note that while all of these diets can have hormone-balancing benefits, it's essential to consult with a healthcare professional to determine which diet is best for you and ensure that you meet your nutritional needs.

The Dairy Effect

When it comes to hormones, dairy products can have a significant impact on your body. Milk contains hormones such as estrogen and progesterone naturally. As these hormones are fat-soluble, they are present in higher levels in whole milk than skim milk. Dairy products also have insulin-like growth factor 1 (IGF-1), which can affect the endocrine system. Consumption of dairy products may increase levels of IGF-1 in the human body, producing androgen hormones such as testosterone, which may worsen hormonal imbalances.

Furthermore, the estrogen in dairy may cause an estrogen overload, leading to problems like weight gain, mood swings, and irregular periods. It can also affect your reproductive system, leading to issues such as endometriosis and breast cancer. Therefore, reducing or eliminating dairy intake may benefit you and your hormonal balance.

It's worth noting that dairy products are not all equal. Yogurt and kefir, two fermented dairy products, contain probiotics that can promote gut health and help maintain hormonal balance. Additionally, dairy products from grass-fed animals may have lower levels of hormones and higher levels of beneficial nutrients like omega-3 fatty acids.

The takeaway message is that consuming dairy products may significantly impact your body's hormonal balance, and it's essential to be mindful of your dairy products. While reducing or eliminating dairy intake may benefit some people, it's crucial to consider the quality and type of dairy products to determine what is best for your hormonal health.

SUGAR ADDICTION ISSUES

Sugar is a highly addictive substance. Someone in your life may have told you more than once that sugar is bad for you. Consuming high amounts of sugar may lead to weight gain, type 2 diabetes, and other health issues. When you eat sugar, it causes a rapid increase in your blood sugar levels, which then leads to a crash, leaving you feeling tired and sluggish. This may create a vicious cycle of constantly needing more sugar to maintain your energy levels and mood. It's important to be aware of your sugar intake and take steps to reduce it if you are consuming more than the recommended maximum amount.

HOW TO STABILIZE YOUR BLOOD SUGAR LEVELS AND ENERGY

Stabilizing your blood sugar levels may help you maintain steady energy levels throughout the day and prevent crashes. Some ways to do this include eating high-fiber foods, such as vegetables, whole grains, and legumes, which slow down the absorption of sugar into your bloodstream. Healthy fats like those in nuts, seeds, and avocados can also help stabilize blood sugar levels. Avoiding processed and sugary foods and beverages and opting for whole, nutrient-dense foods helps keep your blood sugar levels in check.

Shop Healthy to Eat Healthy

One of the best ways to eat healthy is to shop for healthy foods. If you stock your home with healthy, whole foods, you'll be less likely to reach for unhealthy snacks and meals. Some tips for healthy grocery shopping include making a list beforehand, sticking to the store's perimeter, and choosing fresh, whole foods over processed and packaged ones. This can help ensure you get the nutrients you need to support your hormonal balance and improve your health.

Eat Before You're Too Hungry

Skipping meals or waiting until you're overly hungry may lead to blood sugar imbalances and hormonal disruptions. Consuming well-balanced meals at regular intervals during the day can assist in maintaining stable blood sugar levels and preventing sudden drops. Carry healthy snacks with you, such as nuts, seeds, and fresh fruit, to prevent hunger and avoid reaching for unhealthy options when you're on the go.

Avoid Emotional Eating

Many face emotional eating problems that can arise from various emotional triggers such as stress or boredom. Eating to soothe emotions can lead to overeating, weight gain, and disruptions to your hormonal balance. Some tips to avoid emotional eating include identifying triggers, finding alternative coping mechanisms (such as exercise or meditation), and seeking support from friends, family, or a healthcare professional if necessary. By addressing emotional eating and finding healthier ways to cope with emotions, you can support your hormonal balance and overall well-being.

HOW CAN INTERMITTENT FASTING HELP HORMONES?

Intermittent fasting is a dietary approach that involves alternating between periods of eating and fasting. It may significantly impact your hormones by influencing several key hormonal systems in the body, including insulin, growth hormone, and norepinephrine.

- **Insulin:** Intermittent fasting helps reduce your insulin levels and increase insulin sensitivity. Insulin resistance, a significant risk factor for chronic conditions such as cancer, heart disease, and diabetes, can be addressed through this process. By reducing insulin levels and improving insulin sensitivity, intermittent fasting can help regulate blood sugar levels and lower the risk of developing these chronic diseases.

- **Growth hormone:** There is a link between fasting and increased growth hormone secretion. Growth hormone regulates body composition, stimulates muscle growth, and promotes fat loss. Increased growth hormone production may aid in weight loss, muscle gain, and overall health improvement.
- **Norepinephrine:** Intermittent fasting may also help increase the release of norepinephrine. Norepinephrine is a hormone that helps to boost metabolism and promote fat breakdown. Intermittent fasting may help with weight loss and body composition by stimulating the release of norepinephrine.

Overall, intermittent fasting may have a positive impact on hormone levels and help to improve overall health. Intermittent fasting may not be suitable for everyone, especially those with a history of disordered eating or other medical conditions. Fasting may also increase cortisol, a stress hormone, which may lead to overeating or binge eating as it can increase a person's appetite. Knowing the status of your hormones before beginning a diet like intermittent fasting is important.

INFLAMMATION AND THE ENDOCRINE SYSTEM

Inflammation is a natural response of the body to injury or infection. However, it can disturb how the endocrine system should function when it becomes chronic. Chronic inflammation may interfere with the production, release, and metabolism of cortisol, insulin, and thyroid hormones. For example, inflammation can lead to insulin resistance, which can cause the body to produce more insulin to maintain normal blood sugar levels. Over time, this can lead to high insulin levels in the blood, disrupting the production of other hormones and leading to hormonal imbalances.

Symptoms of an Inflamed Body and Gut

These may vary widely depending on the individual and the underlying inflammation causes. Some common symptoms of inflammation in the body include joint pain, stiffness, swelling, fatigue, and fever. Inflammation can also affect the gut, leading to symptoms such as bloating, gas, diarrhea, and constipation. Chronic inflammation in the gut can also disrupt the balance of healthy bacteria in the microbiome, leading to a range of health issues, including hormonal imbalances.

In addition to disrupting the endocrine system's normal functioning, inflammation can lead to other health issues, including heart disease, diabetes, and cancer. Therefore, it's important to take steps to reduce inflammation in the body and promote overall health and well-being.

WHAT ANTI-INFLAMMATORY DIET IS BEST?

An anti-inflammatory diet is a way of eating that can decrease inflammation in the body, leading to improved endocrine systems and hormonal balance. A proper anti-inflammatory diet should consist of whole, unprocessed foods without added sugars, including fruits, vegetables, whole grains, and legumes like beans, fish, poultry, nuts, seeds, and olive oil. Incorporating herbs and spices like cinnamon, ginger, and turmeric into your diet may also be beneficial due to their anti-inflammatory properties.

Heal Your Gut

The gut plays a crucial role in hormonal balance and endocrine function. Inflammation in the gut may disrupt the normal functioning of the endocrine system and affect the production, release, and metabolism of hormones. Identify and eliminate food triggers that may cause gut inflammation. Certain foods can trigger inflammation in the gut, including processed and high-sugar foods, gluten, dairy, and alcohol. Working with a qualified healthcare provider to identify any food sensitivities or intolerances and eliminating trigger foods from your diet may help to reduce inflammation and support gut health.

Gut health is critical to overall health and can impact inflammation levels throughout the body. Incorporating gut-supporting foods into your diet, such as probiotic-rich fermented foods, and taking a high-quality probiotic supplement may support gut health and reduce inflammation.

Increase Intake of Anti-inflammatory Foods

Incorporating more whole, nutrient-dense foods into your diet, such as fresh fruits and vegetables, healthy fats, and lean proteins, may also be helpful. These foods contain compounds that can help to reduce inflammation in the body and support hormonal balance.

Manage Stress

Chronic stress may contribute to gut inflammation, so it's essential to find ways to manage stress in healthy ways. Practices such as meditation, yoga, or regular exercise may help to reduce stress and inflammation in the body, which may support hormonal balance.

WOMEN ACHIEVING BALANCE NATURALLY

There are many stories of women who have achieved hormonal balance naturally. Here are a few examples:

One woman shared her journey of healing Hashimoto's thyroiditis through diet and lifestyle changes. She cut out dairy, soy, and gluten from her diet while increasing the intake of nutrient-dense foods like bone broth, organ meats, and fermented foods. She also addressed stress and sleep issues and gradually reduced her thyroid medication under the guidance of her healthcare provider.

Another woman shared how she manages PCOS (polycystic ovary syndrome) by adopting a low-carb, whole foods diet and incorporating regular exercise. She also addressed her stress levels and worked with her healthcare provider to balance her hormones naturally.

A third woman shared her experience minimizing her endometriosis through dietary changes and natural supplements. She eliminated inflammatory foods like gluten, dairy, and processed foods. She added nutrient-dense foods like leafy greens, bone broth, and wild-caught fish. She also worked with her healthcare provider to address any nutrient deficiencies and imbalances in her hormones.

These stories demonstrate that achieving hormonal balance naturally is possible through dietary and lifestyle changes and working with qualified healthcare providers to address any underlying health issues.

INTERACTIVE ELEMENT

In the spirit of cleaning up your diet, let's get to cooking! Here is an easy, hormone-friendly recipe you can tweak for lunch or dinner, depending on your needs.

Baked Salmon and Broccoli-Black Beans

This healthy baked salmon dish is not just healthy, it is also delicious. Omega-3 fatty acids, which can lessen inflammation and help with hormone synthesis, are abundant in salmon. Broccoli is a good source of fiber, antioxidants, and phytochemicals, which improve liver function and help the body get rid of extra estrogen. Although salmon already contains protein, adding more protein won't hurt as it's necessary to create hormones. Black beans are a high-fiber food, which helps to improve digestion and balance blood sugar levels. This recipe combines the nutritional elements of some everyday superfoods with the comfort of a savory home-cooked meal that is easy to prepare.

Time: 14 minutes

Serving Size: 6

Prep Time: 2 minutes

Cook Time: 12 minutes

Nutritional Facts:

Calories	261
Carbs	9.9 grams
Protein	12.8 grams
Fat	13.4 grams
Sodium	512 milligrams

Ingredients:

- 1 head of broccoli, cut into florets
- 1.5 lbs salmon filet
- 3 garlic cloves, thinly sliced
- 3 tbsp cooked black beans
- 3 tbsp soy sauce
- 6 oz Portobello mushrooms
- 2 tsp sesame oil
- 2 tbsp olive oil

Directions:

- Set oven temperature to 400°F.
- Put the salmon filets on a baking tray and bake until cooked through, about 10 to 12 minutes.
- Meanwhile, heat the olive oil in a pan over medium heat. Throw in the sliced garlic and fry for 2 minutes.
- Add the broccoli and mushrooms to the pan and cook for 3-4 minutes or until tender.
- Stir in the black beans and soy sauce and cook for another minute.
- Spoon the vegetable mixture over the salmon filets, then lightly drizzle with sesame oil.
- If desired, garnish with shredded spring onions.

Your healing journey also involves learning to manage your moods better, so the next chapter gives you practical tips to handle your stress.

CHECKLIST

Day 13

- Journal my symptoms and mood swings.

Day 14

- Make an appointment with my healthcare provider to discuss my concerns about my menstrual cycle or hormonal balance.

Day 15

- Try out the delicious recipe above.

4

DAYS 16 TO 19

MASTERING YOUR MOOD

66 *"The more you worry, the more you throw off the delicate balance of hormones required for health."*

— ANDREW J. BERNSTEIN

D o you worry too much and stress over simple issues? Learn how stress impacts your hormones and uncover effective ways of handling your emotions to improve your overall health.

By the end of this chapter, you'll better understand how to support your body's natural hormone balance and feel more empowered in your journey toward hormonal health.

ONGOING, UNMANAGED STRESS

Experiencing stress is a normal part of life, and your body's stress response system is designed to protect you in times of danger or threat. However, when stress becomes chronic and ongoing, it may lead to adverse health outcomes, including hormone imbalances. This is because the body's stress response system is closely tied to the endocrine system, which produces and regulates hormones.

The key process that controls the body's stress response is the hypothalamic-pituitary-adrenal (HPA) axis. When your body experiences stress, the HPA axis signals the release of the hormone cortisol from the adrenal glands. Remember, cortisol plays a crucial role in the body's stress response. However, when cortisol levels remain elevated due to chronic stress, it may lead to negative health outcomes, including hormonal imbalances.

Unmanaged stress may impact hormone levels in several ways beyond activating the HPA axis. Chronic stress may affect the production and regulation of reproductive hormones, such as estrogen and progesterone, leading to irregular menstrual cycles, fertility issues, and other health concerns. Stress may also impact insulin and glucose regulation, leading to imbalances in blood sugar levels and an increased risk of diabetes.

To manage the impact of stress on hormones, it's important to develop healthy coping mechanisms and stress management strategies.

The Fight-Flight, Sympathetic, and Parasympathetic Systems

The stress response triggers a cascade of physiological and hormonal changes in the body that help prepare you to deal with a perceived threat or danger. The sympathetic and parasympathetic systems are the two branches of the autonomic nervous system, which controls this reaction.

The fight-flight response is triggered by your sympathetic nervous system when it perceives a potential threat or danger. This causes the release of stress hormones such as adrenaline and cortisol, resulting in an elevated heart rate, blood pressure, and breathing rate. These changes help prepare the body to respond quickly to a potential threat.

On the other hand, the parasympathetic nervous system activates the relaxation response, which helps to calm your body down after a stressful event. This system is responsible for slowing the heart rate and breathing, reducing blood pressure, and promoting relaxation.

The balance between these two systems is essential for maintaining overall health and well-being. When the body is under chronic stress, the sympathetic nervous system may become overactive, leading to imbalances in hormone levels and an increased risk of chronic health problems.

Understanding the fight-flight response, the sympathetic, and parasympathetic systems may help you identify when your body is under stress and take steps to activate the relaxation response to promote balance and well-being.

How Can We Manage Our Stress Better?

Self-care is an essential component of maintaining good physical and mental health. It involves taking steps to care for yourself to promote overall wellness, including diet, exercise, sleep, gut health, and hydration. By practicing good self-care, you can support better health and mood.

A critical aspect of self-care is maintaining a healthy diet, which we have already discussed. A diet consisting of whole, unrefined foods with abundant fruits, vegetables, whole grains, lean proteins, and beneficial fats provides the necessary nourishment to energize your body and promote your overall well-being. It's also important to stay hydrated by drinking plenty of water throughout the day.

Regular exercise is another essential component of self-care. Exercise may help reduce stress, boost mood, improve sleep, and support overall physical health. Aim to get at least 30 minutes of moderate exercise most days of the week.

Getting enough sleep is also crucial for good physical and mental health. Aim for 7-8 hours of sleep per night, and establish a regular sleep routine to help support better sleep habits.

Your overall health and well-being can also be affected by the health of the gut. The gut is home to trillions of bacteria that play a vital role in digestion, immune function, and overall health. A fiber-rich diet and probiotic-rich foods like yogurt and kefir can help support a healthy gut.

WHY EXERCISE IS KEY TO HEALTH AND HORMONES?

Regular exercise can profoundly impact your overall health and hormone balance. When you engage in physical activity, you increase blood flow to your muscles and brain, which helps to deliver oxygen and nutrients to these important tissues. Additionally, exercise increases hormone receptor sensitivity, which may help your body respond more effectively to the hormones in your system.

In particular, exercise can significantly impact the levels of hormones like cortisol, insulin, and growth hormone. Physical activity assists in regulating cortisol levels, which may lead to a decrease in stress levels and an enhancement in mood.

When you exercise regularly, your muscles become more sensitive to insulin, which means that your body can better regulate blood sugar levels and prevent spikes in blood sugar.

Exercise may also help increase growth hormone levels in the body, which plays a key role in maintaining muscle mass and bone density. As you age, levels of growth hormone naturally decline, but exercise may help to stimulate the release of this vital hormone.

Exercise for Health Rather Than Weight Loss

We should move our bodies because we love our bodies. Focusing on exercise for health rather than weight loss may lead to several benefits. Exercise may contribute to lowering the risk of various health issues, including diabetes, heart disease, and some forms of cancer. Physical activity may also alleviate stress, improve mental health, and promote healthy sleep habits. Furthermore, research has demonstrated that exercise can enhance general well-being and extend life expectancy (Girdler et al., 2019).

When you exercise for weight loss, there may be a tendency to overemphasize certain types of exercise or push yourself too hard, which may lead to injury or burnout. Focusing on exercise for health instead may help you create a sustainable, long-term exercise routine tailored to your individual needs and goals.

When you exercise for health, it's important to choose activities you enjoy and can realistically maintain over time. This might include walking, swimming, dance, yoga, or strength training. Aim to incorporate various activities into your routine to keep things exciting and challenge different muscle groups.

Keep in mind that physical activity is only a single component of a well-rounded, healthy life. To maximize the benefits of exercise, it's important to focus on other health areas, such as nutrition, sleep, and stress management. Prioritizing overall health and wellness, rather than just weight loss, promotes a more balanced, sustainable approach to exercise and a healthier, happier life overall.

Build a Strong Exercise Habit

It may be challenging to build an exercise habit, especially if you don't enjoy exercising. However, it's essential to incorporate physical activity into your daily routine. Fortunately, there are ways to make exercise more enjoyable and easier to stick to.

Applying behavioral science concepts can assist in creating a regular workout habit. This involves breaking down the habit-forming process into smaller, more manageable steps. For example, start by choosing an activity that you enjoy and scheduling it at the same time each day. Then, gradually increase the duration and intensity of the exercise over time. The key is making the habit small and easy to accomplish.

Finding ways to make physical activity more enjoyable is a different strategy you may employ. This might involve listening to music or a podcast while you work out, exercising with a friend or family member, or trying new activities that you find interesting. By making exercise more fun, you may be more likely to stick with it.

If you hate exercise, it's important to reframe your mindset and focus on its benefits. Instead of thinking of exercise as a chore or punishment, try to view it as a way to improve your health and quality of life. This may involve changing the way you think about exercise and redefining what it means to you.

Another way is having an accountability partner or joining a fitness community which may make a significant difference in keeping you motivated and on track with your exercise goals.

An accountability partner can be anyone you trust to hold you accountable for sticking to your exercise routine. This person can be a friend, family member, or personal trainer. The key is to find someone who is supportive, understanding, and willing to help you stay accountable.

A fitness community can be an excellent source of support and encouragement. Whether it's a fitness class, running group, or gym community, being around like-minded individuals who share similar goals can be motivating and inspiring. These communities can provide a sense of camaraderie and make exercise more enjoyable.

Joining a fitness community provides access to resources and knowledge to help you reach your fitness goals. This may include guidance from experienced fitness professionals, tips for staying motivated, and access to fitness equipment and facilities.

To build a strong exercise habit, it's important to start small and make it a consistent part of your daily routine. This might involve scheduling exercises at the same time each day, setting specific goals and tracking your progress, and finding ways to hold yourself accountable. Over time, the exercise habit will become easier to maintain, and soon enough you'll look forward to the time you spend each day getting stronger.

How Much and What Kind of Exercise Is Best?

The type of exercise you engage in may impact your hormonal balance. As a general recommendation, it's advised to participate in either 150 minutes of moderate-intensity aerobic exercise or 75 minutes of vigorous-intensity aerobic exercise every week. This can be broken down into shorter sessions of 10-30 minutes per day or longer sessions of 45-60 minutes, depending on your preference and schedule (Centers for Disease Control and Prevention, 2022).

Regarding the type of exercise, aerobic exercise (such as running, cycling, or swimming) and strength training (such as weightlifting or bodyweight exercises) have been shown to affect hormone balance positively. Aerobic exercise can help to reduce inflammation, improve insulin sensitivity, and lower cortisol levels. At the same time, strength training can increase testosterone levels and improve insulin sensitivity.

In addition to these types of exercise, engaging in regular physical activity throughout the day is important, such as taking the stairs instead of the elevator or going for a walk during your lunch break. This may increase overall physical activity levels and reduce the time spent sitting, which has been linked to adverse health outcomes.

Overall, balancing aerobic exercise, strength training, and regular physical activity throughout the day can help optimize hormonal balance and improve overall health and well-being. It's essential to consult with a healthcare provider before beginning any new exercise program to ensure that it's safe and appropriate for your individual needs and goals.

GETTING A GOOD NIGHT'S SLEEP

Sleep is essential for maintaining good health and hormonal balance, particularly during menopause and pregnancy, but how much sleep do you need? The amount of sleep a person needs varies based on their age, lifestyle, and individual needs, but the recommended amount of sleep for most adults is between 7–9 hours per night.

Menopause can cause sleep disruptions and insomnia due to hormonal changes, night sweats, and hot flashes. To enhance sleep quality, it's crucial to develop good sleep hygiene, which involves establishing a consistent sleep routine, steering clear of caffeine and alcohol, creating a cozy and cool sleeping environment, and engaging in relaxation methods like meditation and deep breathing.

If you are still having difficulty sleeping despite a solid bedtime routine, speak with a healthcare provider to rule out any underlying medical conditions that may be contributing to your sleep disturbances. Several treatment options are available, including hormone therapy, cognitive behavioral therapy for insomnia, and medication, which can help improve sleep during menopause.

In addition to menopause, other factors that may impact the amount of sleep you need include age, physical activity level, and overall health. Children and adolescents typically need more sleep than adults. Regular exercise may also help improve sleep quality, as long as it's done earlier in the day and not too close to bedtime.

How to Optimize Your Sleep

To optimize your sleep, consider the following tips:

- **Create a comfortable sleep environment:** Ensure your bedroom is conducive to sleep. Keep your bedroom at a comfortable temperature, free from any noise that could disrupt your sleep.
- **Manage light exposure:** Light can disturb your body's natural sleep-wake cycle, so managing your exposure to light is important. Try to get plenty of natural light during the day, and limit exposure to artificial light at night, especially blue light from electronic devices. If you want to control how much light you are exposed to, consider using light-blocking drapes or an eye mask.
- **Get regular exercise:** Frequent physical activity can enhance the quality of your sleep and assist in falling asleep faster.
- **Practice relaxation techniques:** Before bed, try relaxation techniques like deep breathing, meditation, or yoga which can induce a state of calmness in both the mind and body, ultimately leading to improved sleep quality.

- **Invest in a comfortable mattress and pillows:** A good mattress and pillows that support your body can make a big difference in the quality of your sleep.
- **Follow a routine:** Establishing a calming bedtime routine can indicate to your body that it's time to relax and get ready for sleep. This routine can consist of relaxing activities like reading a book, taking a warm bath, listening to soothing music, or practicing relaxation techniques.
- **Limit caffeine and alcohol intake:** Both caffeine and alcohol can interfere with sleep, so it's best to limit your intake, especially in the hours leading up to bedtime. It's also important to remember that some medications and supplements can contain caffeine, so be sure to read labels carefully.
- **Manage stress:** Difficulty falling and staying asleep can be caused by stress and anxiety, so it's crucial to keep your stress levels under control. Engaging in activities such as exercise, meditation, or seeking help from a mental health professional can help manage stress.
- **Melatonin supplements:** Melatonin is a hormone that plays a role in regulating sleep and wake cycles. If you have trouble sleeping or

want to reset your sleep schedule, taking melatonin supplements may be helpful.

- **Use sleep apps:** Numerous sleep apps offer calming sounds, music, or stories to help you drift off. Many offer free trials, so you can experiment with different options until you find one that works for you.
- **Practice meditation or breathing exercises:** Techniques like meditation and controlled breathing may help calm the mind and promote relaxation. To perform the 4-7-8 breathing technique, you need to inhale through your nose for 4 seconds, hold your breath for 7 seconds, and then exhale through your mouth for 8. These practices can help take your mind off of worries about falling asleep.

Set Sleep Schedules

Setting a sleep schedule and routine optimizes your sleep context and improves overall sleep quality. Try to go to bed and get up at the same time every day, including on the weekends, as consistency is important. This will help regulate your body's internal clock and promote better sleep.

Resetting your internal clock can be a helpful strategy for dealing with insomnia. This method involves gradually changing your sleep schedule over several days until you reach the desired bedtime, either by moving your sleep and wake times earlier or later by 15-30 minutes daily. Maintaining consistency and patience throughout the process is essential to allow your body to adjust to the new schedule.

MINDFULNESS PRACTICES

Mindfulness practices like meditation and deep breathing exercises are practical tools to help reduce stress and promote relaxation.

How to Meditate

Meditation is a simple and effective technique that can help you relax and reduce stress. Here are some steps to follow to begin meditating:

- Find a comfy, soothing area to sit or rest.
- Close your eyes and take a few deep breaths to help you relax.
- Focus your attention on your breath. Notice the sensation of the air moving in and out of your body.
- When your thoughts stray, slowly reflect on your breathing. Don't judge or get upset with

yourself for losing focus; bring your attention back to your breath.

- Focus on your breath for several minutes or as long as you like.

As you become more comfortable with meditation, you can try different techniques to help you relax and focus your mind. For example, you can count your breaths, use a mantra or visualization, or observe your thoughts without judgment.

Remember that meditation takes time, determination, and patience to master. Try to meditate regularly, even if it's just for a few minutes each day, and you will likely begin to notice the benefits over time. If self-guided meditation is difficult for you, find one of the many guided meditations available for free online.

How to Do Deep Breathing for Calm

Deep breathing is a simple but effective technique to calm your mind and reduce stress. The benefit of this practice is that you can do it anytime and anywhere.. Here are the steps for doing deep breathing exercises:

- Choose a comfortable and peaceful spot to sit or lie down.
- Put one hand on your chest and the other on your belly.
- Breathe in slowly through your nose, allowing the air to fill your lungs while making sure your diaphragm expands with enough air to stretch your lungs.
- Pause for a few moments while holding your breath.
- Exhale slowly through your mouth, releasing all the air from your lungs.
- Repeat steps three and five for several minutes, concentrating on your breath.

You can also try inhaling through your nose for four counts, then hold your breath for seven. Exhale through your mouth for eight counts, and repeat the cycle for some minutes. Focus on your breath and release any tension or stress in your body.

Both meditation and deep breathing exercises can be incorporated into your daily routine to help reduce stress and improve relaxation. Various apps and guided meditations are also available to help you get started and stay on track with your practice.

MANAGE THE QUALITY OF YOUR THOUGHTS

Managing the quality of your thoughts is essential to maintaining good mental health. Negative self-talk and rumination may be overwhelming and may cause stress and anxiety. To address the quality of your thoughts, you need to be aware of them and identify the patterns that lead to negative thinking. You may practice mindfulness, which helps you observe your thoughts without judgment.

Observing and Reframing Unhelpful Thoughts

Observing and reframing unhelpful thoughts can help you develop a more positive outlook on life. Watching your thoughts makes you more aware of the patterns that lead to negative thinking. This awareness can help you reframe your thoughts and view situations more positively. To reframe unhelpful thoughts, you must challenge the negative beliefs underlying them. You can do this by asking yourself if there is evidence to support your negative beliefs. Often, there isn't, and by recognizing this, you can develop a more positive and realistic perspective.

Learning to reframe unhelpful thoughts takes time and practice. One effective way to do this is through cognitive-behavioral therapy (CBT), which helps you identify and challenge negative beliefs. CBT can be done with a therapist or through self-help techniques. One self-help technique is to use a thought diary, where you write down your negative thoughts and challenge them with evidence-based statements. This helps you recognize the patterns that lead to negative thinking and develop a more positive outlook.

Learn to Identify, Process, and Release Unwanted Emotions

Identifying, processing, and releasing unwanted emotions is important to emotional health. Dealing with negative emotions such as anger, fear, or sadness may be challenging. Still, it's important to take steps to process them in a healthy way. One approach to releasing unwanted emotions is practicing mindfulness and self-awareness, allowing yourself to fully experience the feeling without judgment.

Discussing your feelings and thoughts with someone you trust, such as a close friend, family member, or qualified mental health expert, can be helpful in processing and managing emotions. Additionally, engaging in activities that promote relaxation and stress reduction, such as exercise, meditation, or yoga, can help you manage your emotions more effectively. No single stress reduction technique will fix all of your problems, but each one has its power, and together they give you a full tool chest for building a healthier, happier life.

Releasing unwanted emotions can involve techniques such as deep breathing, journaling, or visualization. By engaging in these practices, you can increase your emotional self-awareness and release negative emotions. It's important to remember that releasing emotions is a process and may take time, but taking steps toward emotional healing can lead to greater well-being in the long run.

Seeking professional help from a therapist or counselor can also be valuable in learning how to identify, process, and healthily release unwanted emotions.

HOW TO CALM DOWN FAST

When experiencing stress or anxiety, knowing how to calm down is essential. Here are some tips to help you calm down fast:

- **Mindful breathing:** The body and mind can be calmed quickly with the 4-7-8 breathing technique. Inhaling through the nose for 4 seconds, holding the breath for 7 seconds, and exhaling with a "whooshing" sound through the mouth for 8 seconds can immediately achieve this effect.

- **Count to 10:** Closing your eyes and counting to 10 slowly will help you to concentrate on something other than your stress.
- **Chew gum:** The slow and methodical act of chewing gum increases blood flow to the brain, helping you to concentrate better and keep a level head during a bout of anxiety.
- **Talk to a friend:** Touching base with someone you love, especially if that person can make you laugh, can provide instant calm. Laughing releases endorphins, which help release tension and elevate the overall mood. In a pinch, a good comedy movie or your favorite goofy laugh-tracked tv show can also lighten the mood.
- **Use lavender:** Aromatherapy, specifically lavender-scented candles or bubble baths, can help alleviate stress and induce relaxation.
- **Cuddle with your pet:** Just 10 minutes of petting your furry friend can reduce stress hormones and promote a feeling of calmness. Don't have a pet? Many animal shelters love volunteers who will pet, wash or brush their animals.
- **Listen to calming music:** Choose calming music with soothing lyrics and rhythm. Singing

along to the music can also help release endorphins.

- **Exercise your body:** Physical activity of any kind helps release stress. You can take a 15-minute break and engage in physical activity like walking briskly, running up and down the stairs, doing a silly dance, or cycling on an exercise bike.
- **Exercise your mind and spirit:** Engage in activities such as yoga, meditation, massage, writing in a journal, giving yourself a pedicure, or taking a soothing nap.

Uncontrolled stress may affect your hormone balance, but many external factors also play a part in hormone balance, and you will discover them in the following chapter.

INTERACTIVE ELEMENT

Managing your thoughts and feelings and understanding how they affect your body is an effective way of managing stress.

Take time each day to reflect on your thoughts and emotions and fill out the thought and mood worksheet below. This will help you identify negative thought patterns and learn how to reframe them positively, leading to a more positive mood and improved hormone balance.

- Write down the situation that triggered your thoughts and emotions.
- In the next column, describe your thoughts about the situation.
- In the third column, write down the emotions and physical sensations you experienced.
- Use the last column to challenge any unproductive thoughts or beliefs contributing to negative emotions.

Difficult Situation	Related Thoughts and Beliefs	Related Emotions and Physical Sensations	Challenge Negativity
Example: Failed interview	*I knew I wouldn't make the cut. I can never succeed.*	Anger, despair, tension in the jaws.	Is it really true that you can never succeed? What could you have done better to win the interview?

CHECKLIST

Day 16

- Assess my stress levels and identify any sources of stress in my life.

Day 17

- Create a self-care routine that includes activities I enjoy and helps me relax.

Day 18

- Consider incorporating mindfulness practices, such as meditation or yoga, into my routine to help reduce stress.

Day 19

- Evaluate my sleep habits and make adjustments as needed to ensure I'm getting enough restful sleep.

Dear Reader,

Thank you for choosing to embark on the transformative journey of hormone balancing with "The Hormone Balancing Revolution for Women." I sincerely hope this book provides valuable insights and practical tools to support your well-being.

If you find "The Hormone Balancing Revolution for Women" to be a valuable resource in understanding your hormones and making positive changes in your life, we kindly request your assistance in spreading the word. Your honest review can make a significant difference in inspiring and empowering other women who may be struggling with hormone imbalances.

By sharing your thoughts and experiences, you can contribute to a community of women seeking support, knowledge, and guidance. Your review can help others make informed decisions about their health and well-being.

Reflect on how "Hormone Balancing for Women" has impacted your life. Has it provided clarity and practical solutions to manage your hormone-related symptoms? Share your personal transformation and how the book has empowered you to take charge of your health. Comment on the comprehensive coverage of topics such as gut health, weight management, and the impact of stress.

Writing a review is a simple yet powerful way to support fellow women on their hormone-balancing journeys. Your feedback will not only assist other readers but also inspire me as an author to continue our mission of empowering women to live their best lives.

We kindly invite you to write a review on Amazon. Your contribution will be greatly appreciated.

Thank you for being a part of this transformative journey. We sincerely value your support, and we look forward to hearing about the positive changes you've experienced as a result of reading " Thormone Balancing Revolution for Women."

Wishing you continued health, happiness, and empowerment!

Warm regards,

Max Hampton

P.S. We appreciate your feedback, whether you have already written a review or are yet to do so. Your thoughts and experiences make a difference in helping others seeking guidance and support.

5

DAYS 20 TO 23

CLEANING UP YOUR ENVIRONMENT

" *"Your genetics load the gun. Your lifestyle pulls the trigger."*

— MEHMET OZ

Have you ever thought that the products you use in your daily life could be affecting your hormones? Taking care of your health involves more than just focusing on your diet and exercise routine. Of all the factors that affect your health, your environment plays an often overlooked, yet crucial role. From the air you breathe to the products you use, your immediate surroundings can impact your hormone balance, mood, and overall well-being. That's why taking a closer look at your environment and adjusting as needed is necessary.

In this chapter, we'll explore some common environmental factors that may significantly impact your health. You can create a cleaner, healthier living space that supports your physical and mental health by making a few changes to your daily habits and routines. So, let's dive in and discover how you can clean up your environment and improve your overall well-being.

ENVIRONMENTAL TOXINS

Exposure to environmental toxins is a growing concern for many people, as it may have adverse effects on the body's delicate hormone balance. Chemicals such as phthalates, bisphenol A (BPA), and dioxins, in particular, are regarded as harmful. These toxins can be found in everyday products like plastics, personal care products, and pesticides, making it difficult to avoid them entirely. Endocrine-disrupting chemicals (EDCs) like phthalates, BPA, and dioxins can cause hormonal imbalances in the body.

Phthalates

Phthalates are a group of chemicals used to soften and increase the flexibility of plastics, making them commonly found in a variety of products, such as a range of health issues, including endocrine disruption. Phthalates can affect testosterone, estrogen, and thyroid hormones. They may also interfere with the adrenal gland's ability to generate hormones such as cortisol and adrenaline. The effects of phthalates on hormone balance may vary depending on the age, sex, and overall health of the individual. Exposure to phthalates has been linked to developmental and reproductive issues in children. In adults, phthalate exposure has been associated with reduced fertility, changes in breast tissue, and increased risk of certain cancers.

Phthalates may enter your body through inhalation, ingestion, and skin contact. Once in your body, they are metabolized and may bind to hormone receptors, activate or block certain enzymes, or alter hormone production and transport. This may lead to changes in hormone levels and signaling leading to the disruption of normal hormone balance. It's imperative to minimize exposure to phthalates whenever possible by choosing phthalate-free products and avoiding products that contain fragrances.

Bisphenol A

BPA is commonly used to produce certain types of plastic, including polycarbonate plastics and epoxy resins. It's also found in some food and drink packaging, as well as in some dental fillings and sealants. Below are some ways in which BPA disrupts hormone balance:

- **Mimicking estrogen:** When Bisphenol A mimics estrogen, it binds to and activates estrogen receptors, leading to hormone levels and signaling changes.
- **Altering testosterone levels:** BPA may also interfere with the production and signaling of testosterone in the body, causing a decrease in your female testosterone levels. This change may negatively affect reproductive health and other aspects of health, such as muscle mass and bone density.
- **Affecting thyroid function:** BPA may also disturb your thyroid, which regulates essential bodily functions, such as metabolism, growth, and development. Disrupting thyroid function may result in various health problems, including weight gain, fatigue, and cognitive impairment.

Minimizing exposure to BPA is vital for maintaining your optimal hormone balance.

Dioxins

Dioxins are very harmful pollutants that are persistent and may be found in several foods, including meat, dairy products, fish, and other seafood. They can also be released into the environment during waste inciner- ation and manufacturing processes.

Dioxins affect several hormones, including estrogen, androgen, thyroid hormones, and corticosteroids. The body's immune, neurological, and reproductive systems may also be impacted.

One way that dioxins disrupt the endocrine system is by binding to and activating the aryl hydrocarbon receptor (AhR), which regulates gene expression and plays a role in various physiological processes, including hormone signaling. When dioxins bind to AhR, they can trigger the production of enzymes that metabolize hormones, leading to their elimination from the body, causing a decrease in hormone levels, which can lead to various health problems.

Dioxins may also interfere with the synthesis and secretion of hormones by disrupting the function of certain enzymes and proteins involved in hormone production. For example, dioxins can inhibit the production of thyroid hormones by interfering with the activity of enzymes involved in iodine metabolism, which is needed to produce thyroid hormones.

Exposure to dioxins may disrupt your body's natural hormonal balance, leading to various health problems, including reproductive and developmental issues, immune system dysfunction, and cancer. It may be beneficial to minimize exposure to dioxins by avoiding or reducing the consumption of high-fat animal products and being mindful of environmental sources of dioxins.

Here is a list of products that may contain phthalates, dioxins, and BPA:

- **Personal care products:** Phthalates are commonly found in personal care products such as fragrances, lotions, deodorants, and hair care products. They may be absorbed through your skin and affect your endocrine system by mimicking the hormone estrogen, leading to reproductive and developmental problems.
- **Plastics:** Some plastics contain phthalates, added to increase their flexibility and durability. These chemicals can be in food packaging, toys, and vinyl floors.

- **Medical devices:** Phthalates may be present in certain medical devices, including blood bags and intravenous tubing.
- **Cleaning products:** Phthalates may be found in some cleaning products, such as detergents and fabric softeners. Exposure to phthalates through inhalation or skin absorption may result in hormonal imbalances.
- **Food:** Phthalates have the potential to transfer from packaging materials into food, especially in high-fat food items.
- **Household items:** BPA may be found in some household items, such as reusable plastic containers and plastic wraps.
- **Food and beverage containers:** BPA is commonly found in plastic food and beverage containers, including water bottles, baby bottles, and the lining of canned foods and drinks.

It's important to note that while not all products contain phthalates, dioxins, or BPAs, they can be found in various everyday products, and exposure to them may lead to health problems. Also, check product labels, research potential sources, and take steps to reduce exposure to these chemicals to minimize their potential negative effects.

HOW TO REDUCE THE RISK?

Reducing the risk of exposure to environmental toxins such as phthalates, bisphenol A, and dioxins can be challenging, but it's possible to take steps to minimize your exposure. One way to do this is by checking the ingredients in your products and making informed choices.

Researching and being aware of what goes into your products is important. Below are some tips to help limit your exposure to harmful substances.

- **Read labels:** Check the ingredient list of household and personal care items and opt for items that do not contain BPA or phthalates. Look for products advertised as BPA-free or phthalate-free, or that employ alternative materials.
- **Use glass or stainless steel:** Use glass or stainless steel containers to store food and beverages instead of plastic containers, especially for hot liquids or high-fat foods.
- **Avoid plastic wrap:** To cover food, substitute wax paper or aluminum foil for plastic wrap.
- **Choose fresh foods:** Eat fresh foods instead of canned or processed foods, as these are more likely to contain BPA.

- **Use natural cleaning products:** Choose natural cleaning products that do not contain phthalates or other harmful chemicals.
- **Grow your food:** Consider growing your food using organic methods, which reduces the need for pesticides and herbicides.
- **Ventilate your home:** Make sure your home is well-ventilated to reduce the concentration of airborne toxins.

Keep in mind that even little changes can have enormous effects. Taking the initiative to reduce exposure to harmful chemicals helps protect your hormone balance while promoting your overall health.

Make Your Cleaning Detergents

Cleaning products are essential to maintain a clean and healthy home environment. However, many conventional cleaning products contain harmful chemicals that may adversely affect your health and the environment.

Making your cleaning detergents gives you control over the ingredients used. That way, you can ensure the products are safe for you and the environment. Homemade cleaning products are often more affordable and customizable, allowing you to create products that cater to your cleaning needs.

In the following sections, you will learn how to make your own general polish, polish cleaner, and washing detergent using simple ingredients you may already have in your home. If you prefer unscented personal care items and cleaning supplies, just omit the essential oils from the recipe in the following sections.

▷ General Polish

This recipe is great for polishing wood furniture, stainless steel appliances, and other hard surfaces. The olive oil helps to condition and protect the surface, while the vinegar helps to clean and remove dirt and grime.

Ingredients:

- 18 drops of preferred essential oil
- ½ cup pure olive oil
- ½ cup white vinegar

Instructions:

- Pour the white vinegar into a spray bottle and mix with the olive oil.
- Add the essential oil, then gently shake until the polish blends well.

- Spray onto furniture or other surfaces and use a soft cloth to polish.

▷ Lavender Polish Cleaner

This recipe is excellent for cleaning and polishing glass and mirrors. The rubbing alcohol helps to remove fingerprints and smudges, while the vinegar helps to clean and shine the surface. The cornstarch helps to reduce streaking.

Ingredients:

- 1 tbsp cornstarch
- ½ cup rubbing alcohol
- 11 drops lavender or preferred essential oil
- ½ cup white vinegar

Instructions:

- In a spray bottle, mix the white vinegar, rubbing alcohol, and cornstarch, then add the lavender or another essential oil of your choice.
- Shake well to mix the cleaner.
- Spray onto surfaces and use a soft cloth to polish.

▷ Soaps

Here's a recipe for making homemade soap. Working with lye can be dangerous and requires proper safety precautions, such as wearing gloves and eye protection. It's essential to follow the recipe carefully and avoid contact with the lye solution.

Ingredients:

- 1 lb coconut oil
- 21 drops preferred essential oil
- 1 lb olive oil
- 32 fl oz water
- 1 lb palm oil
- 13 oz lye

Instructions:

- Combine the oils in a slow cooker or use a large pot.
- Set the heat to low and heat them until they melt.
- Using a separate bowl, weigh the lye, then mix it with the water. Gently stir until it dissolves.
- Add the lye solution to the melted oils, then use a stick blender or a hand blender to mix the

soap mixture for about 30 minutes or until you get a pudding-like consistency.

- Add the essential oil, pour the soap mixture into molds, and cover with a towel.
- Leave it to cure for 4-6 weeks, occasionally turning it to ensure even curing.
- Cut the soap into bars and store it in a cool, dry place.

▷ Washing Detergent

This recipe makes about 32 ounces of detergent, which should last approximately 32 loads. When you want to use it, scoop 2-3 tablespoons of the detergent per load of laundry.

Ingredients:

- 1 cup washing soda
- 26 drops of preferred essential oil
- 1 cup borax
- 1 bar grated castile soap

Instructions:

- Mix the borax and washing soda in a large bowl.
- Combine the mixture with the castile soap and mix well.
- Add your preferred essential oil for fragrance.
- Store the washing detergent in an airtight container.

Make Your Own Beauty Products or Buy Ones You Have Researched

In today's world, it's becoming increasingly important to be mindful of the ingredients in the products you use on your body. Commercial beauty products contain various chemicals and additives that may harm your health and well-being.

Making your beauty products or purchasing ones you have thoroughly researched may help you avoid harmful ingredients and promote a healthier lifestyle. By doing so, you'll have greater control over what you put on your body and reduce your exposure to potentially dangerous chemicals. In addition, making your beauty products can be a fun and rewarding experience that allows you to customize products to your preferences and needs.

Whether you're looking to avoid harmful ingredients or want to try something new, making your beauty products or carefully selecting ones to purchase can be a great choice. Below we will look at some recipes for beauty products and self-care items that will make you feel crafty, pampered, and healthy. Let's get started, then.

▷ Face and Body Creams / Lotions

Here is a recipe for a homemade face and body cream or lotion free of harmful chemicals. You can customize this recipe using different base or carrier oils and essential oils depending on your skin type and preferences. Lavender is a scent that can aid in sleep and relaxation. For a more energetic scent, try sweet orange or mint essential oils.

Ingredients:

- ¼ cup jojoba oil
- 13 drops of lavender essential oil
- ½ cup shea butter
- 1 tsp vitamin E oil
- ¼ cup sweet almond oil
- ½ cup coconut oil

Instructions:

- Melt the coconut oil and shea butter over low heat in a heat-safe bowl or double boiler.
- Switch the heat off and let the melted mixture cool for some minutes.
- Add the vitamin E, almond, lavender, and jojoba oil to the cooled mixture and stir until all ingredients combine well.
- Prepare a clean container or glass jar and pour the mixture into it.
- Leave the mixture for a few hours so it completely cools and solidifies.
- After it solidifies, use a stand or hand mixer to whip the mixture until it becomes light and fluffy, which may take several minutes.
- Transfer the whipped mixture to a final container and store it in a cool, dry place. Your cream or lotion should last for several months.

▷ **Body Wash**

Here's a recipe for making your own body wash free of harmful chemicals. This body wash recipe is gentle on the skin, making it suitable for most skin types. However, if you have sensitive skin or are prone to allergies, it's always best to test the product on a small area of the skin before using it all over your body.

Ingredients:

- 1 tbsp vegetable glycerin
- ¼ cup honey
- 13 drops of lavender essential oil
- ¼ cup jojoba oil
- 1 cup distilled water
- 1 cup castile soap

Instructions:

- Combine the honey, castile soap, lavender, and jojoba oil, in a mixing bowl and blend them well.
- While continuously stirring to combine, slowly add the distilled water to the mixture.
- Add the vegetable glycerin to the mixture and stir well for a thicker body wash, but omit it if you want your body wash lighter.
- Prepare a container with a lid, or an empty bottle you like, then pour the mixture into it.
- Gently shake the bottle before each use so that all the ingredients mix well.
- To use, apply your body wash to wet skin and rinse thoroughly with water.

▷ Shampoo

Here's a recipe for a simple homemade shampoo. This shampoo won't lather as much as commercial shampoos, but it will still effectively cleanse your hair. Depending on your hair type, you may need to adjust the amount of honey or oil.

Ingredients:

- 7 drops of lavender essential oil
- ¼ cup liquid castile soap
- 1 tsp coconut oil or olive oil
- ¼ cup water
- 1 tsp honey

Instructions:

- Combine the water, castile soap, and oil in a small jar or bowl.
- Stir well, add the honey, and stir until well mixed.
- Add the lavender or your preferred essential oil.
- Transfer the shampoo into a clean jar with a lid, or use a bottle.
- To use, wet the hair and massage a small amount of shampoo into your scalp and hair. Rinse well with warm water.

Creating your own beauty products can be an enjoyable and satisfying process. It enables you to manage what components are included in your products and may save you money. However, it's essential to research and ensure you're using safe and effective ingredients. Always patch-test new products before using them all over your face or body, and consult with a healthcare professional if you have any concerns.

Use Organic Pesticides

Using organic pesticides may be beneficial for both your health and the environment. Organic pesticides are made from natural ingredients such as plants, minerals, and oils, and they are often safer to use around children, pets, and wildlife than synthetic pesticides. Organic pesticides break down more quickly and do not leave toxic residues in the soil or water.

Unlike their organic counterparts, non-organic pesticides are usually derived from synthetic chemicals that can harm your health and the environment. These pesticides can remain in the environment for extended periods, building up in soil, water, and organisms. Exposure to non-organic pesticides has been linked to various health problems, including cancer, congenital disabilities, and neurological disorders.

One of the main differences between organic and non-organic pesticides is their composition. Organic pesticides are made from natural substances that are generally considered safe. In contrast, non-organic pesticides are made from synthetic chemicals that may have toxic effects, which can affect your hormones and may be a risk factor for developing certain cancers.

Organic pesticides are also typically used in lower quantities. They are more targeted, reducing the risk of unintended harm to beneficial insects, birds, and other organisms. Furthermore, organic farming methods typically encourage natural pest management through crop rotation, planting companion crops, and using beneficial insects, which can help decrease the dependence on pesticides.

Below are some tips that may help you use organic pesticides effectively.

- **Identify the pest:** Before choosing a pesticide, knowing what you're dealing with is essential. Identifying the pest will help you select the most effective organic pesticide.
- **Choose the right pesticide:** Once you've identified the pest, choose an organic pesticide designed to target that specific pest. There are many different types of organic pesticides, so

choosing the right one for your needs is important.

- **Follow instructions carefully:** Carefully read the instructions on the pesticide label and follow them closely. Some organic pesticides may need to be diluted before use, and others may need to be applied at a particular time of day or in a specific way.
- **Be persistent:** Organic pesticides may take longer to work than chemical pesticides, so it's essential to be patient and persistent. You may need to apply the pesticide more than once to achieve the desired results.
- **Use protective gear:** Even though organic pesticides are generally safer than chemical pesticides, it's still important to protect yourself while using them.

Organic pesticides protect your plants and crops without harming you, your family, or the environment. Always read the label and pay close attention to the instructions to guarantee the most efficient and secure usage.

Only Buy Plastic Containers That Are Rated Environmentally Friendly and Food-Safe

Choosing plastic containers that are rated environmentally friendly and food-safe over traditional or non-food-safe plastics may benefit the environment as well as your health. Food-safe plastics are tested and approved by regulatory agencies such as the FDA (Food and Drug Administration) and the EU (European Union) to ensure they are safe for food storage and packaging. These plastics are made without harmful chemicals that can leach into your food or beverages and disrupt your hormonal balance.

On the other hand, non-food-safe plastics, especially those made with Bisphenol A (BPA) or phthalates, can mimic the effects of hormones in the body and lead to hormonal imbalances. These chemicals can interfere with the body's endocrine system and disrupt the normal functioning of hormones, leading to various health problems such as infertility, obesity, and cancer.

These plastics are also better for the environment because they are made from sustainable materials and can be recycled or reused. They're also made to be biodegradable, lessening the amount of garbage in landfills and the ocean.

When choosing plastic containers, look for ones labeled as food-safe and free of harmful chemicals such as BPA and phthalates. These containers are frequently composed of polyethylene materials, such as high-density polyethylene (HDPE), low-density polyethylene (LDPE), polypropylene (PP), or polyethylene terephthalate (PET), and are regarded as safe for contact with food.

Overall, using environmentally friendly and food-safe plastics is vital in promoting a healthier and more sustainable lifestyle. Reducing exposure to harmful chemicals and supporting eco-friendly practices can improve your overall well-being and contribute to a healthier planet.

Cut Back on Plastics in the Home

Cutting back on plastics in the home can benefit both the environment and your health, particularly in reducing exposure to harmful chemicals that can affect your hormones. Here are some ways to cut back on plastics in the home:

- Consider using glass containers rather than plastic ones to store food and drinks. Glass is a safe and non-toxic material that doesn't release harmful chemicals into your food or beverage.

- Opt for reusable water bottles made from stainless steel, glass, or other non-plastic materials to avoid exposure to potentially harmful chemicals. Disposable plastic water bottles can release toxic substances, especially when exposed to high temperatures or sunlight.
- Avoid using plastic utensils, plates, and cups. Instead, choose wood, bamboo, stainless steel, or glass options.
- Use cloth or reusable bags for grocery shopping instead of single-use plastic bags.
- Look for plastic-free alternatives for personal care and household items, such as bamboo toothbrushes, wooden hairbrushes, and natural fiber cleaning cloths.
- Buy pads and tampons without plastics, fragrances, or bleach, or use a menstrual cup or washable, reusable pad.

Reducing our reliance on plastics lessens our exposure to harmful chemicals and lowers plastic pollution in our environment.

We have established that cleaning up your environment can substantially impact your hormone balance and overall health. Minimizing exposure to harmful chemicals in typical household and personal care products may be all you need to reduce the risk of hormone-related health issues. With a little effort and awareness, creating a healthier environment for yourself is possible.

There are many mainstream medicines and natural supplements you can try out to help ease hormonal imbalances. The next chapter explores the options you have for treating hormonal imbalances.

CHECKLIST

Day 20

- Take inventory of my household cleaning, personal care, and gardening products to identify potentially harmful chemicals and ingredients.

Day 21

- Research alternative, more natural options for these products and start replacing them as needed.

Day 22

- Consider switching to organic produce and meats to reduce exposure to hormone-disrupting pesticides and antibiotics.

Day 23

- Pay attention to changes in my hormone balance and adjust my routine as needed.

6

DAYS 24 TO 28

PILLS AND PANACEAS

> *"Medicine is not only a science; it's also an art. It does not consist of compounding pills and plasters; it deals with the very processes of life, which must be understood before they may be guided."*
>
> — PARACELSUS

When struggling with hormonal imbalances, the search for relief can be daunting. Many turn to traditional Western medicine, while others seek out alternative therapies. Both approaches have their merits and drawbacks. Conventional medicine offers potent pharmaceuticals and scientifically proven treatments, but it also comes with side effects and a focus on treating your symptoms rather than the root cause.

Alternative therapies, on the other hand, emphasize a holistic approach to health and wellness but may lack the same level of scientific evidence and regulation.

In this chapter, we will explore both options and provide insights into various treatments for hormonal imbalances. While providing you with this information, I encourage you to take a thoughtful and informed approach in considering your options and work closely with a trusted healthcare professional to create a personalized treatment plan that works for you.

THE PROS AND CONS OF WESTERN MEDICINE AND HORMONE THERAPY

Many alternatives are available for addressing hormonal abnormalities, including conventional medicine and hormone therapy. Although these methods may help treat symptoms, they also have possible dangers and disadvantages that must be considered. To help you choose your course of treatment, we will weigh the benefits and drawbacks of hormone therapy and Western medicine in this section.

Pros of Western Medicine and Hormone Therapy

Hormone therapy can effectively alleviate symptoms associated with hormonal imbalances, such as hot flashes, night sweats, mood swings, and sleep distur-bances. In addition, there are several other benefits associated with hormone therapy, such as a reduced risk of osteoporosis and bone fractures, improved mental well-being, decreased tooth loss, lower risk of colon cancer and diabetes, modest improvement in joint pains, and lower death rates for women who begin hormone therapy in their 50s.

The evidence-based approach of Western medicine is a significant advantage in hormone therapy. Hormone therapy has been studied for decades and is backed by a vast body of research. The hormones used in hormone therapy are carefully selected, and their dosages are precisely controlled to ensure maximum safety and efficacy.

Hormone therapy is a valuable tool for managing hormonal imbalances, particularly for conditions such as menopause, hypothyroidism, and low estrogen levels. Postmenopausal women who undergo hormone replacement therapy (HRT) may experience a decreased risk of bone fractures, heart disease, and stroke. HRT may also relieve menopausal symptoms such as hot flashes, night sweats, and vaginal dryness.

Furthermore, hormone therapy is often a critical component of cancer treatment. Some malignancies, including female breast cancer, are largely influenced by hormones in their development and progression. Hormone therapy may be used to suppress hormone production or block the hormones' effects on cancer cells, effectively slowing or stopping tumor growth.

Overall, the evidence-based approach of allopathic medicine and hormone therapy may provide a safe and effective treatment option for managing hormonal imbalances and related conditions. However, as with any medical treatment, weighing the potential benefits against the risks and discussing them with a healthcare provider to determine the best course of action is essential.

Cons of Western Medicine and Hormone Therapy

Side Effects

While effective in treating hormonal imbalances, it may also have drawbacks. One notable drawback is the possibility of adverse effects, including breast tenderness, fluid retention, nausea, and headaches. Additionally, hormone therapy may increase the risk of certain health conditions, such as blood clots, stroke, and breast cancer. Other potential side effects include bloating, mood changes, vaginal bleeding, and skin irritation. Regular monitoring by your healthcare provider is crucial to ensure that any negative effects are detected and managed promptly. Please note that not everyone will experience the same side effects.

Cost

One major drawback of Western medicine and hormone therapy is the cost. Hormone therapy can be expensive, especially if not covered by insurance. In addition to the cost of the hormones themselves, additional costs may be associated with doctor visits, lab tests, and follow-up appointments. If you do not have insurance coverage or have limited financial resources, the cost of hormone therapy may be prohibitive. This can lead to a lack of access to treatment, which may negatively affect your health and well-being.

Alternative Options

Alternative therapies such as herbal supplements, acupuncture, or dietary changes may be preferred by some people instead of hormone therapy. These options can be less expensive and have fewer side effects. However, they may not be as effective as hormone therapy for some individuals. It's important to note that the effectiveness of alternative treatments varies and may not have the same level of scientific evidence as hormone therapy. Additionally, getting medical advice before implementing alternative treatments is critical.

COMMON MEDICATIONS FOR HORMONE IMBALANCES

Hormone Replacement Therapy for Perimenopausal and Menopausal Symptoms

By now, you know that hormone replacement therapy (HRT) is a medication commonly used to alleviate perimenopausal and menopausal symptoms. HRT is typically prescribed if you have been experiencing peri or postmenopausal symptoms. HRT works by supplementing your body's natural hormone levels with synthetic hormones.

There are two types of HRT: estrogen-only therapy (ET) and combined estrogen-progestin therapy (EPT). ET is a good option if you have had a hysterectomy and no longer have a uterus, while EPT is recommended if you still have a uterus. EPT contains both estrogen and progestin to reduce the risk of uterine cancer.

While HRT may effectively reduce menopausal symptoms, it is not a long-term solution. HRT is associated with an increased risk of certain health conditions, including blood clots, stroke, and breast cancer. You may not be a suitable candidate for HRT if you have a history of these health conditions.

You may also experience side effects from HRT, including breast tenderness, nausea, and bloating. HRT is associated with an increased risk of developing gallbladder disease and urinary incontinence.

Despite these risks and side effects, many women continue using HRT longer than recommended. Some women may not be aware of the risks associated with long-term HRT use. In contrast, others may find that the benefits of HRT outweigh the potential risks. You must have open and honest discussions with your physician about HRT's potential benefits and risks and carefully consider your options before deciding.

Thyroid Hormone Replacement Therapy

Thyroid hormone replacement therapy is a standard treatment for hypothyroidism, which hinders your thyroid gland from producing enough thyroid hormone. Levothyroxine, a synthetic form of the thyroid hormone, is most frequently used for thyroid hormone replacement treatment.

The side effects of this form of HRT are generally mild but may include tremors, increased heart rate, and insomnia. To avoid developing hyperthyroidism, a disease in which your thyroid gland generates too much thyroid hormone, it's advisable to work with your doctor to find the correct medication dosage.

This form of HRT is typically a lifelong treatment because hypothyroidism is a chronic condition. Regular blood tests are needed to monitor thyroid hormone levels and adjust medication dosages as needed.

While thyroid hormone replacement therapy may effectively manage hypothyroidism, you can also consider other alternative treatments such as dietary changes, supplements, or herbal remedies. Be sure to discuss any alternative therapies with your physician before starting because they may interfere with the effectiveness of thyroid hormone replacement therapy.

Hormonal Birth Control

Using synthetic hormones to prevent pregnancy is the primary purpose of hormonal birth control. These hormones prevent ovulation and modify the cervical mucus, making it more challenging for sperm to reach and fertilize an egg. Hormonal birth control may also assist in regulating menstrual cycles and reducing symptoms associated with conditions like PCOS.

Changes in menstrual bleeding are a frequently observed side effect of hormonal birth control, which can manifest as lighter or heavier bleeding, spotting, or irregular bleeding. Hormonal birth control may also result in other side effects like breast tenderness, nausea, headaches, and mood swings. Although rare, hormonal birth control can increase the risk of blood clots, stroke, and heart attack, particularly in women who smoke or have other risk factors.

Using hormonal birth control is not suitable for everyone. Certain medical conditions, such as high blood pressure or a history of blood clots, may make it impossible to use these drugs.

Glucocorticoids

Glucocorticoids are a medication commonly used to treat adrenal insufficiency, in which the adrenal glands are not producing enough cortisol. As you recall, cortisol is an important hormone that helps regulate your body's response to stress and helps maintain blood sugar levels, among other functions. Glucocorticoids, such as hydrocortisone, are synthetic versions of cortisol that supplement the body's natural cortisol production.

While glucocorticoids can effectively manage adrenal insufficiency, they can also have significant side effects. These can include weight gain, high blood pressure, osteoporosis, muscle weakness, increased risk of infection, and mood changes. Long-term use of glucocorticoids may also increase your risk of developing diabetes, cataracts, and other conditions.

Aromatase Inhibitors

Aromatase inhibitors are a class of medications used to treat estrogen-dependent conditions, such as breast cancer. They block an enzyme called aromatase, which converts androgens into estrogen. This reduces estrogen levels in the body, which can slow the growth of certain types of breast cancer.

Although aromatase inhibitors have shown efficacy in breast cancer treatment, they may result in adverse reactions. Joint pain, hot flashes, vaginal dryness, and bone loss are typical side effects. In uncommon situations, aromatase inhibitors may lead to severe complications such as heart issues, liver impairment, and osteoporosis.

Gonadotropin-Releasing Hormone (GnRH) Analogs

Gonadotropin-releasing hormone (GnRH) analogs can potentially treat health issues associated with reproductive hormones, including uterine fibroids and endometriosis. These medications work by suppressing the production of hormones in the ovaries, which can help alleviate symptoms.

Some common examples of GnRH analogs include leuprolide (Lupron), goserelin (Zoladex), and nafarelin (Synarel). These medications are usually administered by injection or nasal spray.

Similar to other medicines, GnRH analogs may lead to some side effects. These can include reduced sex drive, mood swings, hot flashes, headaches, and vaginal dryness. Long-term use of GnRH analogs may also increase the risk of osteoporosis and bone fractures.

It's important to discuss the potential benefits and risks of GnRH analogs with your doctor before starting treatment. In some cases, other medicines or management options may be more appropriate.

Key Micronutrients for Hormone Rebalancing

Maintaining a healthy diet and adequate nutrition may significantly affect hormone balance. Certain micronutrients, or vitamins and minerals, may support the production and regulation of hormones in your body. This section will discuss some crucial micronutrients for hormone rebalancing and how they can be incorporated into a healthy diet.

Magnesium

Magnesium is essential in many bodily functions, including muscle and nerve function, bone health, and immune system regulation. It's also important for hormone health and may be especially helpful in hormone rebalancing. Magnesium has numerous benefits for thyroid health, helping to regulate thyroid function and reducing the symptoms of an underactive thyroid. Additionally, magnesium has a calming effect on your body, making it helpful in managing stress and promoting better sleep.

One of the critical benefits of magnesium for hormone health is its ability to support the production of your main sex hormones, which include estrogen, progesterone, and testosterone. Magnesium also helps the liver metabolize hormones and excrete harmful estrogen metabolites, which may help prevent hormone imbalances.

Various magnesium supplements, such as magnesium citrate, magnesium glycinate, magnesium oxide, and magnesium chloride, can be found. Each type has a different level of absorption and effectiveness.

Magnesium citrate is commonly used for its ability to support bowel regularity and ease constipation. The body easily absorbs magnesium glycinate, which can promote relaxation and improve sleep. Magnesium oxide is inexpensive and commonly used for its laxative effects. Magnesium chloride is easily absorbed, supporting healthy immune function and reducing inflammation.

Iodine

If you want to support your thyroid health, ensuring you're getting adequate iodine in your diet is essential. One primary nutritional trigger for hypothyroidism is insufficient iodine, a necessary mineral for producing thyroid hormones.

The average recommended daily intake for adults is 150 micrograms per day, and many food sources of iodine can help you meet this goal. Some of the best sources of iodine include seaweed, fish, dairy products, and iodized salt. Iodine is present in fruits, vegetables, and grains in smaller quantities.

If you're concerned about your iodine intake or think you may have a thyroid condition, it's essential to talk to your healthcare provider. They can help you determine if you need to increase your iodine intake or if there are other steps you can take to support your thyroid health.

Selenium

Consuming adequate selenium will promote the health of your thyroid. Selenium is a mineral that aids in producing thyroid hormones in your body and has anti-inflammatory antioxidant qualities. Taking 200 mg of selenium daily as a supplement may lessen thyroid antibodies and elevate mood.

Zinc

Zinc is a vital mineral that has a significant role in regulating and producing hormones. It helps transform cholesterol into progesterone, which is necessary for keeping up healthy estrogen and testosterone levels. Zinc is also essential in creating thyroid hormones; a zinc deficiency can result in hypothyroidism.

To ensure you get enough zinc, consuming 5-15 mg of zinc daily is best. The best way to obtain zinc is through your diet, and some excellent sources of zinc-rich foods include oysters, beef, chicken, beans, nuts, and whole grains. Zinc supplements can also be an option, but it's always best to get your nutrients from whole food sources whenever possible.

Probiotics and Probiotic Foods

Gut health plays an important role in balancing your hormones because the gut is responsible for metabolizing and secreting hormones and producing neuro-transmitters that may impact hormonal balance. The gut is also home to trillions of microorganisms, including beneficial bacteria that help to maintain a healthy gut microbiome. An imbalance in the gut microbiome, known as dysbiosis, can lead to inflammation, insulin resistance, and impaired hormone metabolism. This can lead to endocrine problems like estrogen dominance and adrenal exhaustion.

One way to support your gut health is by consuming probiotics through probiotic supplements or probiotic-rich foods. Probiotics are live microorganisms that help promote the growth of healthy gut bacteria, which can improve digestion and overall gut health.

Foods naturally rich in probiotics include fermented foods such as sauerkraut, kimchi, kefir, and yogurt. Consuming these foods regularly can help maintain a healthy balance of gut bacteria and improve hormone balance.

It's also necessary to eat prebiotic-rich foods. Prebiotics are fibers that your body can't break down. They feed the good bacteria in your gut, which helps them grow and stay healthy. Foods rich in prebiotics include garlic, onions, asparagus, bananas, and chicory root. Consuming probiotic and prebiotic-rich foods can help support your gut health and promote hormone balance.

Herbal Supplements

Herbal supplements are plant-based products that are used to promote health and wellness. They come from herbs, roots, leaves, flowers, and other plant materials. Herbal supplements have been used for thousands of years in traditional medicine. They are still popular today as a natural alternative to traditional medicine. They come in various forms, such as teas, capsules, extracts, and powders, and are used to support various aspects of health, including hormonal health. In this section, we will list some herbal supplements and how they may help you alleviate some hormonal imbalances.

- **Black Cohosh:** This plant is frequently used to relieve symptoms related to menopause, such as hot flashes, vaginal dryness, and night sweats. It is thought to help balance hormone levels by interacting with serotonin receptors in the brain and reducing the secretion of luteinizing hormone (LH) from the pituitary gland.
- **Vitex agnus-castus:** Also known as chaste tree, this herb is mainly used to control menstruation, lessen PMS symptoms, and boost fertility. It works by stimulating the pituitary gland to increase the secretion of luteinizing hormone (LH) and reduce the secretion of

follicle-stimulating hormone (FSH), which helps to balance progesterone and estrogen levels.

- **Dong Quai:** Often referred to as the "female ginseng," Dong Quai regulates menstrual cycles and alleviates menstrual cramps. It contains phytoestrogens, which are believed to mimic the effects of estrogen in the body and help to balance hormone levels. The herb has also been used to treat hot flashes and mood changes from menopause.
- **Ashwagandha:** This herb is commonly used in Ayurvedic medicine to reduce stress and anxiety. It works by reducing cortisol levels in the body, which can help to balance hormone levels.
- **Passionflower:** Primarily used to reduce anxiety and promote relaxation, passionflower may also improve sleep quality, which can help balance your hormone levels. It works by increasing the levels of gamma-aminobutyric acid (GABA) in the brain, which can help to reduce stress and anxiety.
- **Milk thistle:** This plant is often used to help the liver stay healthy and eliminate toxins. It makes the liver make more glutathione, a powerful antioxidant that protects the liver

from damage. Milk Thistle also has anti-inflammatory properties that can help reduce inflammation and keep hormone levels in balance.

- **Zizyphus:** Commonly used in traditional Chinese medicine to promote relaxation and improve sleep quality, this herb also has antioxidant properties. It may help reduce inflammation in the body and balance hormone levels. The herb works by increasing the levels of GABA in the brain, which can help to reduce stress and anxiety.

Always consult a healthcare professional before starting any herbal supplement, especially if you are pregnant, breastfeeding, or have a medical condition. Also note that the FDA does not regulate herbal supplements and should be used with caution, as they can interact with medications and cause side effects.

Aromatherapy Oils for Hormones

Aromatherapy oils are natural plant extracts used to promote physical and emotional well-being. These oils are often used in conjunction with massage, inhalation, or other therapeutic techniques to help balance hormones and alleviate various symptoms associated with hormonal imbalances. When used correctly, aromatherapy oils can have a powerful effect on the body and mind, helping to reduce stress, improve mood, and support overall health and well-being. Ingesting essential oils may be dangerous and is not advised. Some essential oils can be harmful if applied to the skin. Consult an expert and always follow the directions when using essential oils.

The following is a list of aromatherapy oils for hormones:

- **Clary sage:** This essential oil may alleviate menstrual cramps, PMS symptoms, and hot flashes. It has a soothing impact on the nervous system, which can lessen stress and encourage relaxation.
- **Frankincense:** An excellent choice for reducing inflammation in your body.
- **Thyme:** This oil's antimicrobial effects may aid in the prevention of illnesses. Thyme also helps control menstruation and alleviate PMS symptoms.
- **Lavender:** If you struggle with menstrual cramps, this essential oil promotes relaxation, potentially reducing stress and improving sleep. It also has pain-relieving properties and may help other symptoms of PMS.

- **Rosemary:** This oil has a stimulating effect on the nervous system, which can help to improve concentration and memory.
- **Peppermint:** Struggling with menopause symptoms? The cooling effect of peppermint is what you need for your hot flashes. The oil may also aid in reducing menstrual cramps and other PMS symptoms.
- **Rose:** This essential oil has a calming effect on the nervous system and can help to reduce stress and anxiety.

How to Use the Oils

You can use aromatherapy oils in a variety of ways to support hormonal health. One common way to use essential oils is inhalation, either through a diffuser or by adding a few drops to a bowl of hot water. As you may have noticed in some recipes covered earlier, you can even use essential oils in your house products. Topical application may involve adding a few drops to a carrier oil and applying it to the skin. You can also incorporate oils into bathwater or use them during a massage.

It's important to consult with a healthcare professional before using essential oils, especially if you are pregnant or have any underlying health conditions.

- **In your bath:** To unwind and relax, add essential oils to your bath water. Firstly, add a few drops of the essential oil you prefer to a carrier oil or Epsom salt in a cup, then put it into the bathwater.
- **Burner:** You can also use a diffuser or burner to spread the fragrance of essential oils into your environment. Place a few drops of the essential oil into the water in a diffuser or burner.
- **In your lotions:** You may also mix them with your lotions or creams. Add a few drops of your preferred essential oil to a carrier oil such as almond or coconut, and then mix it with your lotion or cream. Afterward, apply it to your skin.

Before using essential oils on your skin, always dilute them with a carrier oil and test an essential oil on a small area of the skin first.

We have discussed various treatment options for hormonal imbalances, including pharmaceuticals and herbal supplements. It's important to remember that your body is unique, and what works for someone you know may not work for you. Next, let's establish strong routines to support a healthier lifestyle. Adopting a positive mindset and a happy lifestyle starts with you!

INTERACTIVE ELEMENT

▷ *Turmeric-Ginger Tea*

Turmeric and ginger are known for their anti-inflammatory properties, which can help reduce inflammation and promote hormone balance. Here's how to make turmeric-ginger tea:

Ingredients:

- 1 tsp fresh lemon juice
- 1 tbsp grated fresh ginger
- 4 cups water
- 1 tbsp grated fresh turmeric

Directions:

- Boil the water, then add ginger and turmeric.
- Reduce the heat and simmer the tea mixture for 14 minutes.
- Switch the heat off, then let the tea steep for another 5 minutes.
- Mix in the lemon juice, strain the tea into a cup, and enjoy!

▷ *Chaste Tree Berry Tea*

Chaste tree berries are a popular herb for women's health because they contain compounds that help balance hormones. Here's how you make it!

Ingredients:

- 1 tsp dried red raspberry leaves
- 1 tsp honey
- 1 tbsp dried chaste tree berries
- 4 cups boiling water
- 1 tbsp dried dandelion root

Directions:

- Combine the dried chaste tree berries, dandelion root, and red raspberry leaves in a pot with boiling water.
- Lower the heat and leave the tea to simmer for 16 minutes.
- Remove the pot from the heat and let the tea steep for another 4 minutes.
- Strain the tea into a cup, then add some honey.

▷ *Raspberry Leaf Tea*

Raspberry leaf is an excellent ingredient for hormone balance because it contains fragarine, a compound that helps to regulate estrogen levels in the body.

Ingredients:

- 1 tsp dried lemon balm leaves
- 1 tsp honey
- 1 tbsp dried raspberry leaves
- 4 cups water
- 1 tsp dried oat straw
- 1 tsp dried nettle leaves

Directions:

- Mix the dry tea ingredients in a pot with boiling water.
- On medium to low heat, simmer the tea for 15 minutes.
- Switch off the heat and leave the tea to steep for about 5 minutes.
- Strain the tea into a cup, add honey, and enjoy!

CHECKLIST

Day 24

- Research different treatment options for hormone imbalances and discuss them with my healthcare provider.

Day 25

- Explore integrative therapies such as acupuncture, massage, and meditation for natural symptom relief.

Day 26

- Make more dietary changes such as reducing sugar and processed foods and increasing intake of whole, nutrient-dense foods.

Day 27

- Incorporate regular exercise into my routine, such as strength training and cardio.

Day 28

- Prioritize stress management techniques such as journaling, mindfulness, and spending time in nature.

7

DAYS 29 TO 33

MAKING BALANCE A WAY OF LIFE

> *"Never underestimate the power you have to take your life in a new direction."*

— GERMANY KENT

Wouldn't you love to create healthy habits that stick? You can build a healthy routine that supports your hormone health with just a few changes!

To maintain a healthy hormonal balance, adopting healthy habits and making them a consistent part of your lifestyle is paramount. This means establishing a routine that supports your physical, mental, and emotional well-being. In this chapter, we'll explore the importance of finding meaning and motivation in your wellness journey and how to build strong routines that will help you maintain balance in all areas of your life.

HOMEOSTASIS

It is all about balance.

The ability of the body to maintain a stable internal environment despite changes in the external environment is called homeostasis. This physiological mechanism is essential for optimal body functioning and health maintenance. Examples of homeostasis in the body include controlling blood sugar levels, maintaining a constant body temperature, and regulating heart rate and blood pressure. A detailed example of how homeostasis is achieved in your body is through temperature regulation.

The average temperature of your body is between 97 and 99 degrees Fahrenheit. When the body's temperature fluctuates outside this range, it could significantly negatively affect your health. To avoid this, the hypothalamus in the brain serves as the body's thermostat to keep your body temperature in balance. It collects information from temperature receptors spread out throughout the body and then sends instructions to different organs to start reactions that either increase or decrease the generation of body heat.

Let's say your body temperature increases over the average; the hypothalamus will cause the sweat glands to release perspiration, which will evaporate and cool your skin. It will also enhance blood circulation to the skin, stimulating heat release through radiation. The hypothalamus will instruct the muscles to relax, making it simpler for heat to escape via the skin. Now let's say you are feeling cold; your hypothalamus will cause you to shiver, which produces heat by increasing muscular activity. To prevent heat loss via the skin and maintain warm blood circulation to the internal organs, the hypothalamus will also send instructions that will help restrict blood vessel size.

With that example, you might think that you have no control over this balance called homeostasis because your body will balance everything automatically. Actually, you have an important part to play in all this.

Homeostasis is achieved through various factors such as diet, hydration, activity, sleep, and hormones. Each of these factors plays a crucial role in maintaining your body's internal environment within a narrow range of parameters, despite changes in the external environment.

What Can Happen if Homeostasis Is Disturbed?

Disrupting homeostasis may cause various health problems and diseases, such as:

- **Chronic diseases:** When your body cannot maintain hormonal balance, it may lead to chronic diseases such as diabetes, heart disease, and hypertension.
- **Hormonal imbalances:** The endocrine system is mainly responsible for maintaining homeostasis. If the endocrine system is malfunctioning, this may lead to various medical conditions, which we have looked at already.
- **Poor immune system:** Homeostasis is crucial in supporting the immune system. When homeostasis is disrupted, the immune system can weaken, making it more difficult for the body to fight infections and diseases.
- **Mental health issues:** The maintenance of homeostasis also has an impact on the brain and nervous system. When the balance is disturbed, it can result in mental health problems like depression and anxiety.

You may play an active role in achieving homeostasis by maintaining a healthy lifestyle. This includes eating a balanced diet, staying hydrated, engaging in regular physical activity, getting enough sleep, managing stress levels, and avoiding harmful substances such as tobacco and excessive alcohol.

EVERYDAY HABITS AND ROUTINES AFFECT YOUR HORMONES

You already know by now that your body has a complex endocrine system that produces hormones, which regulate various bodily functions, and that hormones play a vital role in your overall health and well-being, including regulating your sleep, metabolism, mood, and reproductive functions. However, many everyday habits and routines may disrupt your hormone balance, negatively affecting your health. So, what are these daily habits, and how do they affect your hormones?

- **Hydration:** Hormone regulation depends on staying hydrated since it helps control body temperature, blood pressure, and the movement of hormones throughout the body. Dehydration can reduce the production of several hormones, including vasopressin and aldosterone, resulting in electrolyte imbalances and other problems.

- **Sleep:** Lack of sleep or irregular sleep patterns may interfere with your hormone production of cortisol, insulin, and melatonin, which may lead to weight gain, insulin resistance, and unpredictable sleep-wake cycles.

- **Exercise:** Regular exercise may help keep your hormones in check by reducing insulin resistance, encouraging the release of endorphins, and controlling cortisol levels.

- **Diet:** Consuming a well-balanced diet high in protein, good fats, and complex carbs will help to regulate blood sugar levels, lessen inflammation, and support good gut flora. In turn, these effects may assist in controlling hormones, including estrogen, cortisol, and insulin.

- **Stress management:** Stress causes the production of cortisol to rise while the production of other hormones like estrogen and progesterone falls. Lowering cortisol levels and balancing hormones can be achieved by engaging in stress-reduction practices, including yoga, meditation, and deep breathing.

The science underlying these effects is intricate and involves several pathways, including the gut-brain axis and the HPA axis (hypothalamic-pituitary-adrenal axis). Chronic stress, inadequate sleep, and other variables have been shown to alter the HPA axis, which plays a critical role in controlling stress hormones like cortisol. The gut-brain axis, influenced by nutrition, stress, and inflammation, refers to the two-way communication between the gut and the brain. This axis regulates hormones like insulin, leptin, and ghrelin, controlling appetite and energy balance.

Establishing a new routine is essential to creating healthier habits, particularly when achieving hormone balance. Putting new choices into daily practice is an effective way to make them a part of your lifestyle. This is because routines and habits are deeply ingrained in our brains, and repetition is the key to forming new habits. Developing a new routine trains your brain to associate healthy habits with certain triggers, making them easier to implement.

HOW DO WE ESTABLISH A NEW ROUTINE?

Even though establishing a new routine may be difficult, with the appropriate attitude, it's possible to make it a good habit for you. Below are some clues that may help you establish a new routine.

- **Identify the new habit you want to establish:** The first step is to determine what new habit you want to incorporate into your daily routine. Be specific about what you want to achieve and how you want to do it. For instance, if you're going to incorporate exercise into your daily routine, specify the time, place, and type of exercise.

- **Set realistic goals:** The next step is to set realistic and achievable goals. Start with small goals that can be easily accomplished, and gradually increase the intensity or frequency of the habit. This will encourage you to keep going by giving you a sense of success and helping you gain momentum.

- **Plan your routine:** Once you have identified the new habit and set realistic goals, it's time to plan your routine. Think about what time of day you want to do the habit and how long you want to spend on it. Create a schedule that fits into your daily routine and stick to it.

- **Start small:** Starting small helps to build momentum and makes it easier to stick to your new routine. Begin with small, manageable tasks such as doing five minutes of meditation per day or going for a 10-minute walk.

- **Stay consistent:** The secret to creating a new routine is consistency. Make a conscious effort to stick to your plan and commit to your new habit. Consistency helps to build momentum and makes it easier to turn your new habit into a routine.

- **Eliminate obstacles:** Identify any barriers preventing you from sticking to your routine and find ways to eliminate them. For example, if you have trouble waking up early to exercise, try going to bed earlier, or lay out your workout clothes the night before.

- **Stay accountable:** One of the most significant factors in establishing a new routine is accountability. Find ways to hold yourself accountable, such as using a habit tracker or telling a friend about your new routine. This can aid in maintaining your motivation and staying focused.

- **Be patient and persistent:** It takes time to establish a new routine, and there will be setbacks along the way. Be patient with yourself and stay persistent. Don't give up if you miss a day or two; refocus and get back on track.

- **Reward yourself:** Recognize and celebrate your accomplishments, and reward yourself for your hard work. Celebrating your progress helps to keep you motivated and makes it easier to stick to your new routine.

HOW TO MAKE LIFESTYLE CHANGES THAT STICK

Before you learn how to make lifestyle changes, you need to know how to make the brain function to adapt to changes.

Developing a behavior involves the creation of new neural pathways in your brain, which are strengthened over time with repetition and reinforcement. The brain is a complex network of neurons that communicate with each other through synapses, which are the connection points between them. When you repeat a behavior, the neurons involved in that behavior become more connected, and the synapses between them become stronger. The ability of the brain to change and adapt throughout one's life is referred to as neuro-plasticity.

Repetition is critical in developing a new behavior because it strengthens the neural pathways associated with it. When a behavior is repeated, the neural pathway associated with it becomes more efficient, which makes it easier for you to perform the behavior in the future. By increasing the chances of behavior repetition, reinforcement plays a crucial role in developing a new behavior. Positive reinforcement, such as rewards, can help to strengthen the neural pathways associated with the behavior. In contrast, negative reinforcement, such as punishment, can weaken those pathways.

It's worth noting that the brain is naturally inclined to pursue pleasure and evade pain. Therefore, behaviors associated with pleasure, such as eating tasty food or engaging in enjoyable activities, are more likely to be repeated. On the other hand, behaviors associated with pain or discomfort, such as exercising when you are out of shape, are less likely to be repeated, but with consistency, your brain will adapt to these behaviors.

Developing a new behavior involves creating and strengthening neural pathways in the brain through repetition and reinforcement. By understanding the science behind behavior development, we can use this knowledge to develop and stick to new habits and behaviors.

The Habit Loop

Another way to change a lifestyle is by understanding and taking advantage of the habit loop. What is a habit loop?

The habit loop describes how your brain creates and maintains habits. Each habit comprises three parts: the cue, routine, and reward. The cue is the initial trigger that prompts the pattern to begin. This can be anything, such as a particular hour of the day or location. A habit itself, which may be mental or physical action, is the routine. The benefit of a happy feeling that results from finishing the routine is the reward. The habit loop creates a neurological connection between the cue and the reward, with the routine acting as the bridge. The more times we complete the routine and receive the reward, the stronger the connection becomes until the habit's automatic and effortless.

You may develop new habits that stick if you incorporate the habit loop. You may create a routine and link it to a reward that reinforces the behavior by finding a particular cue that causes the desired action. For instance, if you want to start exercising more frequently, you can set a schedule for exercising at a specific time each day as your cue. Reward yourself with a nutritious snack or a calming activity afterward.

The new behavior becomes established in your brain by constantly following the habit loop, which makes it simpler to maintain and less likely to vanish over time. And just like that, you have made lifestyle changes that you may stick to.

HOW TO GET CLEAR OF YOUR LIFESTYLE VALUES

Getting clear on your lifestyle values is essential to making sustainable changes in your life. Understanding the "why" behind the changes you want to make is necessary. Doing so will clarify what you hope to gain from those changes. Here are some tips on how to get clear on your lifestyle values.

- **Determine your core values:** Core values are the fundamental beliefs or ideals you consider the most important guiding principles in your life. They guide your behavior, decisions, and actions, as explained above. Identifying your core values will help you understand what is most important to you and what you want to achieve.

- **Self-reflection:** Take time to reflect on what is most important to you. What do you value the most? What brings you the most happiness and fulfillment? What are your passions and interests? Consider writing down your thoughts and feelings.

- **Prioritizing:** After you have outlined your principles and identified what's important to you, prioritize these values. What is your top priority? What values come next? Listing your core principles will help you maintain focus on your priorities.

- **Alignment:** Examine how your current lifestyle aligns with your goals, priorities, and beliefs. Are there areas of your lifestyle that conflict with your targets or values? What changes can you make to align your life with your principles?

- **Action:** Once you clearly understand your values and how they align with your lifestyle, take action to make changes that will bring your life into better alignment with your values. This may involve creating new habits or routines, setting goals, or making other changes to help you live a more fulfilling and authentic life.

- **Create a list of goals:** Make a list of goals consistent with your fundamental values after you have determined what they are. When you have a clear understanding of your goals, you will be able to prioritize your time and energy effectively.

- **Understand your motivation:** Understanding your reason for making changes in your life will help you stay committed to your goals.

Motivation can come from a variety of sources, including personal values, desires, or beliefs.

- **Identify potential obstacles:** Before making changes, identify any obstacles that may hinder your progress. By identifying these obstacles, you can develop a strategy to solve them.

- **Evaluate your progress:** Regularly evaluate your progress as you start making changes. This will help you identify what is working and what is not. You can then adjust your approach accordingly.

- **Seek support:** Getting support from friends, family, or a professional can help you stay committed to your goals. One of the best motivators is having someone hold you responsible.

Getting clear on your lifestyle values is essential to making lasting changes in your life. Now that you have the tools to support your hormone balance and overall well-being let's go through some inspiring stories from other women who have been on this journey before.

INTERACTIVE ELEMENT

A vision board can be a powerful tool for manifesting your goals and dreams, including a healthy and hormone-balanced approach to life. Below is a simple method to create one that's hormone-friendly!

- Start with a clear intention. Before you begin, think about what you want to achieve with your hormone-balanced lifestyle. You may want to improve your sleep, increase your energy, or reduce your stress levels. Write down your intention and keep it in mind as you create your vision board.
- Gather your materials. You will need a poster board or cork board, magazines, scissors, glue, and markers. Look for images and words that represent your intention and hormone-balanced lifestyles, such as healthy foods, exercise, relaxation, and self-care.
- Create your layout. Arrange your images and words on the board in a way that feels visually appealing and inspiring to you. You can organize them by theme, color, or any other way that feels right.
- Personalize it. Add personal touches that reflect your individuality and unique journey. You may

want to include a photo of yourself or a quote that inspires you.

- Display it prominently. Hang your vision board in a place where you will see it every day, such as your bedroom or office. Take a few moments each day to look at it and visualize yourself living your hormone-balanced lifestyle.

Remember, a vision board is not a magic wand but can be a powerful reminder of your goals and aspirations. Focusing on your intention and taking action towards a hormone-friendly lifestyle gives you room for a healthier, more balanced life.

CHECKLIST

Day 29

- Analyze my daily routine and identify areas where I can make healthier choices for my body and hormones.

Day 30

- Implement a consistent sleep schedule and prioritize getting enough quality sleep each night.

Day 31

- Incorporate regular physical activity into my routine, whether through structured exercise or simple lifestyle changes like taking the stairs instead of the elevator.

Day 32

- Experiment with self-care practices, such as relaxing baths or practicing mindfulness, to find what works best for me.

Day 33

- Consider working with a healthcare provider or hormone specialist to help me develop a personalized plan for hormone balance and overall health.

8

REAL WOMEN SPEAK UP

> *"All truth passes through three stages. First, it's ridiculed. Second, it's violently opposed. Third, it's accepted as being self-evident."*

— ARTHUR SCHOPENHAUER

It may be challenging to know what to do with so much conflicting information online and armchair experts everywhere you look. However, understanding these myths and the truth behind them is essential for effectively managing hormone imbalances. In this chapter, we will discuss some top myths about hormone imbalances and why they are wrong, then discover stories from others' experiences. Some incredible women allowed me to share their stories with you so you'd know you aren't alone.

MYTHS ABOUT HORMONE IMBALANCES

Many people believe that hormone imbalances only occur during menopause. However, hormone imbalances can occur at any age and every gender can experience them.

Although thyroid disorders are more frequently diagnosed in women, they can also occur in men. It's a common misconception that only women can be affected by thyroid disorders. The likelihood of men developing a thyroid disorder is one in eight during their lifetime.

Hormone imbalances can cause various health issues, such as mood swings, weight gain, and fatigue.

Dispelling myths about hormone imbalances is crucial for effectively managing these health issues. It fuels you to seek accurate information from credible sources and consult healthcare professionals for personalized advice.

SURVIVING INTENSE PERIODS DURING PERIMENOPAUSE

Perimenopause is when a woman's body begins to transition into menopause. This transition is marked by changes in hormonal levels that can cause a range of symptoms, as you will discover in Lizzy's story below.

"I never thought I'd be one of those women who sit around and complain about their periods all the time, but when perimenopause hit, it was like a whole new world of craziness. My periods became erratic, with heavy bleeding one month and nothing the next. I was also dealing with hot flashes, night sweats, and mood swings that made me feel like a hormonal teenager all over again.

One day, I found myself in the grocery store, crying over a head of lettuce. Yes, lettuce, you read correctly! The fact that it was the final one on the shelf made me feel like everything was working against me. I knew I needed to get a handle on my hormones and fast.

I started researching and realized that my diet had a huge role in my hormonal imbalance. I cut out processed foods and started eating more whole foods, like leafy greens and lean protein. I also got personalized treatment options and started taking supplements to help regulate my hormones.

Slowly but surely, my symptoms started to improve. I wasn't crying over lettuce anymore, and my periods were becoming more regular. It was like a miracle! Of course, there are still days when my hormones feel like they are all over, but now I know how to manage it. And if all else fails, there's always chocolate." —Lizzy

Lizzy's story teaches us the importance of understanding our bodies and seeking personalized treatment options for hormone imbalances and perimenopause. Remember, perimenopause and menopause are not the end of the world. It's just the start of a new chapter filled with crazy mood swings and the occasional urge to throw rotten lettuce at someone's head. With the right mindset, information, and support, you can face your hormones and tell them to stay under control.

THE TRUTH ABOUT WEIGHT, WOMEN, AND HORMONES

Hormones are crucial in regulating metabolism, appetite, and weight in women. As you age, hormonal changes can affect your weight gain and make it more challenging to lose weight if you don't address your hormonal imbalance.

"When I was trying to lose weight, I did all the things books and posts talk about—eating right, exercising, and more. But nothing worked. Not a pound, not half.

After countless blogs and journals, I started to realize that my hormones could be the culprit. I came to understand that imbalanced hormones can make weight loss more challenging. I thought, "Great, just what I need—another obstacle in my weight loss journey!"

But I'm not one to give up easily, so I decided to get my hormones checked. That's when I discovered that my estrogen levels were way too high. No wonder my body is holding onto every extra pound!

I could have gone the traditional route and just popped some hormone pills. Realistically though, who wants to cope with such adverse effects? Not me. I looked into natural ways to balance my hormones, then changed things such as drinking green tea, adding flaxseed to my diet, and even getting more sunlight.

After some time, the scale started moving in the right direction, and my clothes could fit better. And the best part? The good old-fashioned natural remedies saved me from relying on crazy pills and fad diets."—Megan

Megan's story shows that hormone imbalances can sabotage weight loss efforts. Getting hormone levels checked and seeking natural remedies to balance hormones is effective in aiding weight loss.

MENOPAUSE MISFORTUNE

Menopause marks the end of a woman's reproductive life. It is caused by the natural decline in reproductive hormones, mainly estrogen. It affects a woman's health and well-being, including mood, sleep, and weight. Hormonal imbalances during menopause can cause many symptoms, from hot flashes and night sweats to mood swings, depression, anxiety, and more. Managing menopausal symptoms requires a holistic approach that may include lifestyle changes, medication, and hormone replacement therapy.

"I was in my late forties when I started experiencing the symptoms of menopause. Night sweats and mood swings had become my new normal. I was also struggling with weight gain and a general feeling of sluggishness that I couldn't shake.

I turned to my doctor, hoping for some relief. But all he could offer was hormone replacement therapy, which I wasn't keen on. I started doing research and stumbled upon a website dedicated to helping women balance their hormones naturally.

Their approach was refreshing—they emphasized the importance of diet, stress management, and gentle exercise rather than just popping pills. I started following their advice and was amazed at the results. Within weeks, my hot flashes had decreased, my mood had improved, and I was even starting to shed some of the extra weight.

The website offers a variety of resources, including articles, recipes, and even a 7-day hormone reset program. I found the recipes especially helpful; they were easy to follow and delicious, and they incorporated hormone-balancing ingredients, such as leafy greens and healthy fats."—Sandy

Sandy's experience strengthens the point that there are natural ways to manage menopause symptoms and that a one-size-fits-all approach is not always the answer. With the right tools and support, you can take charge of your health and live your best life, even amid menopause.

OVERCOMING CHRONIC FATIGUE AND HORMONAL IMBALANCES

Chronic fatigue and hormonal imbalances can profoundly impact a woman's quality of life, often causing exhaustion, mood swings, and other disruptive symptoms. While traditional medical approaches may provide adequate relief, holistic and integrative therapies can give hope and some real solutions.

"My success story knocked people's socks off when I shared my journey in a support group one evening. My hormones were all over the place, and I'll admit, I was a hot mess!

But then, I discovered a wellness institute that turned my life around. They looked at my hormones like they were a math equation to be solved, and they actually figured out how to balance them out.

They took a holistic approach to my health, looking at my lifestyle, diet, and hormone levels. They found that I had high cortisol levels and estrogen dominance, which were causing my symptoms. The first step was to adjust my diet and lifestyle habits. They helped me cut out sugar, caffeine, and processed foods and then ensured I incorporated more fruits, vegetables, and whole foods into my diet.

The institute also recommended that I start practicing yoga and meditation to help manage my stress levels. Adding to these lifestyle changes, they prescribed me a customized hormone therapy plan, which included bioidentical hormone replacement therapy (BHRT) and supplements to help balance my hormones.

After a few weeks of following this plan, I started to notice significant improvements in my mood, energy levels, and overall well-being. Once my hormones were in check, everything fell into place, and I even lost some weight."—Elsa

Elsa's story shows that getting a comprehensive view of your health is imperative to address the root cause of your symptoms and find the right tools and support for your unique situation.

You know you are not alone. Countless women have gone through similar journeys and come out stronger, healthier, and happier on the other side. The stories you've read in this chapter are just a few examples of the incredible transformations possible when you prioritize your health and take control of your hormones. So, don't give up. Keep going and know that you have the power to create the life and body you want.

THE DAMAGE HORMONES CAN DO

Lastly, I'd like to tell Cassie's story. Her journey was a rollercoaster of emotions, filled with pain, sadness, and frustration. At 37, she had been diagnosed with PCOS after years of uncontrolled hormonal imbalances from the time she was at university. Her diagnosis was devastating, but the news that she had also become infertile was the final straw. Cassie had always dreamt of becoming a mother, but now, that dream was shattered. The misery that came with her pressure to conceive cost her everything- her job, marriage, and self-worth.

For months, Cassie lived in a dark hole of depression, feeling hopeless and alone. It wasn't until she reluctantly joined a support group that things started changing. Being able to share her story with other women going through the same thing was just the revelation she needed. She realized she wasn't alone and that there was hope.

With the help of her new friends and a great therapist, Cassie began her journey toward healing. She took charge of her health by seeking treatment for PCOS, making lifestyle changes, and focusing on a healthier diet. It wasn't easy, but she knew she had to take control of her life, and I respect that about her.

Once she was sure her recovery was going well, Cassie began exploring other options for becoming a mother. She looked into adoption and found a beautiful baby boy who continues to light up her life. She moved to a new town, asked her mother to move in with her, and they became a happy family.

Now, Cassie runs a support group, helping other women struggling with hormone imbalances and infertility. She knows firsthand how hard it can be, but she also agrees that reclaiming your life and finding joy is possible. Cassie's journey reminds us that we all have the strength to overcome adversity and that hope is always within reach.

CONCLUSION

As you come to the end of this book, I hope you have gained valuable insights and inspiration on your journey to balancing your hormones. Achieving hormone balance is an ongoing journey that requires dedication, patience, and a willingness to make changes to your lifestyle. You have what it takes to become your best advocate and take charge of your healing process. By being better informed, asking lots of questions, and being open to trying new options, you stand a good chance of creating a better hormone and health profile. So, take that first step and commit to a healthier and more balanced life.

Remember, your body is unique; what worked for someone you know may not work for you. The key is to listen to your body, be patient with yourself, and seek out the support and guidance you need. I hope this book has empowered you to take charge of your health and provided you with practical tools to create lasting change.

Dear Reader,

We hope you've enjoyed reading "The Hormone Revolution for Women" and found it to be a valuable resource in your hormone-balancing journey. As we approach the end of this transformative book, we kindly remind you of the power of sharing your thoughts and experiences.

We would greatly appreciate it if you could take a moment to review "The Hormone Revolution for Women" on Amazon. Your honest feedback can make a significant impact on other readers seeking guidance and support in their own hormone-balancing endeavors.

By leaving a review, you contribute to a community of women empowering one another to take charge of their health. Please consider sharing your insights, the impact the book has had on your life, and any positive changes you've experienced as a result.

Thank you for being a part of this revolution and for considering to review "The Hormone Revolution for Women" on Amazon. Your support means the world to us.

With sincere appreciation,

Max Hampton

P.S. Your review can help inspire and guide other women on their hormone-balancing journeys. We are grateful for your time and for sharing your thoughts.

REFERENCES

Acme, K. (2022, August 3). *The ultimate guide to food-grade and food-safe plastics*. Acme Plastics. https://www.acmeplastics.com/content/the-ultimate-guide-to-food-grade-and-food-safe-plastics/

Ali, S. A., Begum, T., & Reza, F. (2018). Hormonal influences on cognitive function. *Malaysian Journal of Medical Sciences, 25*(4), 31–41. https://doi.org/10.21315/mjms2018.25.4.3

Anderson, E., & Zagorksi, J. (2022, February 28). *Probiotics & prebiotics*. Center for Research on Ingredient Safety. https://www.canr.msu.edu/news/probiotics-prebiotics-foods

Anthony, K. (2017, October 13). *High testosterone levels in women*. Healthline; Healthline Media. https://www.healthline.com/health/high-testosterone-in-women

Barcal, L. (2022, October 5). *3 ways to make your own beauty products*. https://www.wikihow.com/Make-Your-Own-Beauty-Products

Barrea, L., Pugliese, G., Laudisio, D., Colao, A., Savastano, S., & Muscogiuri, G. (2020). Mediterranean diet as medical prescription in menopausal women with obesity: A practical guide for nutritionists. *Critical Reviews in Food Science and Nutrition, 61*(7), 1201–1211. https://doi.org/10.1080/10408398.2020.1755220

Baton Rouge clinic. (2021, January 7). *How to calm down fast*. Baton Rouge Clinic. https://batonrougeclinic.com/how-to-calm-down-fast/

Bernhard, B. (2022, October 25). *What to know about low testosterone (low T) in women*. EndocrineWeb. https://www.endocrineweb.com/conditions/low-testosterone/low-testosterone-in-women

Bernstein, A. J. (n.d.). *Andrew J. Bernstein quotes*. BrainyQuote. Retrieved April, 2023, from https://www.brainyquote.com/quotes/andrew_j_bernstein_499415?src=t_hormones

Better Health Channel. (2012). *Obesity and hormones*. https://www.

betterhealth.vic.gov.au/health/healthyliving/obesity-and-hormones

Britannica. (2018). *Homeostasis.* https://www.britannica.com/science/homeostasis

Cahalan, S. (n.d.-a). *Susannah Cahalan quotes.* BrainyQuote. Retrieved April, 2023, from https://www.brainyquote.com/quotes/susannah_cahalan_929362?src=t_hormones

Carlyle, T. (n.d.). *Thomas Carlyle quotes.* BrainyQuote. https://www.brainyquote.com/quotes/thomas_carlyle_118220

Centers for Disease Control and Prevention. (2021, June 29). *Creating a good sleep environment.* Centers for Disease Control and Prevention. https://www.cdc.gov/niosh/emres/longhourstraining/environment.html

Centers for Disease Control and Prevention. (2022, June 2). *How much physical activity do adults need?* Centers for Disease Control and Prevention. https://www.cdc.gov/physicalactivity/basics/adults/index.htm

Childs, W. (2021, October 12). *The best form of zinc to take for your thyroid.* https://www.restartmed.com/the-best-form-of-zinc-to-take-for-your-thyroid/

Chu, M. (2016, July 28). *The 3 stages of truth in life.* HuffPost. https://www.huffpost.com/entry/the-3-stages-of-truth-in_b_11244204

Clean Sweep Effect. (2022, January 17). *16 essential oil cleaning recipes.* https://www.cleansweepeffect.com/16-essential-oils-cleaning-recipes/

Clear, J. (2018, November 13). *How to start new habits that actually stick.* James Clear. https://jamesclear.com/three-steps-habit-change

Cleveland Clinic. (2021a, January 12). *Does what you eat affect your mood?* Health Essentials from Cleveland Clinic. https://health.clevelandclinic.org/bad-mood-look-to-your-food/

Cleveland Clinic. (2021b, December 10). *Cortisol: What it is, function, symptoms & levels.* Cleveland Clinic; Cleveland Clinic. https://my.clevelandclinic.org/health/articles/22187-cortisol

Cleveland Clinic. (2021c, December 16). *Insulin Resistance: What It Is,*

Causes, Symptoms & Treatment. Cleveland Clinic. https://my.cleve landclinic.org/health/diseases/22206-insulin-resistance

Cleveland Clinic. (n.d.). Inflammation: *What is it, causes, symptoms & treatment*. Cleveland Clinic. Retrieved April 28, 2023, from https://my.clevelandclinic.org/health/symptoms/21660-inflammatio

Corinne O'Keefe Osborn. (2017, December 18). *Everything you should know about hormonal imbalance*. Healthline. https://www.healthline.com/health/hormonal-imbalance

Cronkleton, E. (2019, September 9). *How to use essential oils with a diffuser, on the skin, in a bath, more*. Healthline. https://www.health line.com/health/how-to-use-essential-oils

Daly, T. (n.d.). *Tess Daly quotes*. BrainyQuote. Retrieved April, 2023, from https://www.brainyquote.com/quotes/tess_daly_1192780?src=t_hormones

Davidson, K. (2020, February 5). *Mood food: 9 foods that can really boost your spirits*. Healthline. https://www.healthline.com/nutrition/mood-food

Day, J. (2020, January 29). *Estrogen dominance & progesterone deficiency*. The Holland Clinic. https://thehollandclinic.com/perimenopause/estrogen-dominance-progesterone-deficiency/

Duckworth, K. L. M. (2018, May 1). *Using behavioral science to build an exercise habit*. Scientific American. https://www.scientificamerican.com/article/using-behavioral-science-to-build-an-exercise-habit/

Earley, B. (2021, March 24). *Stuck in a rut? Consider making a vision board*. Oprah Daily. https://www.oprahdaily.com/life/a29959841/how-to-make-a-vision-board/

Fletcher, J. (2019, February 12). *4-7-8 breathing: How it works, benefits, and uses*. Medical News Today. https://www.medicalnewstoday.com/articles/324417

Flynn, H. (2022, November 1). *Intermittent fasting: What is its impact on hormones?* Medical News Today. https://www.medicalnewstoday.com/articles/does-intermittent-fasting-affect-female-hormones

Gabriel, C. (2020, February 19). *11 of the best foods for hormone balance*. HUM Nutrition Blog. https://www.humnutrition.com/blog/best-foods-for-hormone-balance/

Germaine. (2020, August 24). *3-Ingredient hormone balancing tea recipe for women*. Live Well Zone. https://livewellzone.com/hormone-balancing-tea-recipe/

Girdler, S. J., Confino, J. E., & Woesner, M. E. (2019). Exercise as a treatment for schizophrenia: A review. *Psychopharmacology Bulletin, 49*(1), 56–69. https://www.ncbi.nlm.nih.gov/pmc/articles/PMC6386427/

Gore, A. C., Chappell, V. A., Fenton, S. E., Flaws, J. A., Nadal, A., Prins, G. S., Toppari, J., & Zoeller, R. T. (2015). EDC-2: The Endocrine Society's Second Scientific Statement on Endocrine-Disrupting Chemicals. *Endocrine Reviews, 36*(6), E1–E150. https://doi.org/10.1210/er.2015-1010

Griffin, R. M. (2009, December 4). *Hormone replacement therapy*. WebMD. https://www.webmd.com/menopause/guide/hormone-replacement-therapy#1

Gunnars, K. (2019, March 7). *The 8 most popular ways to do a low-carb diet*. Healthline; Healthline Media. https://www.healthline.com/nutrition/8-popular-ways-to-do-low-carb

H, the D. experts of T. F., & Magazine, yman. (2023, March 20). *How to make homemade cleaner with simple ingredients*. Family Handyman. https://www.familyhandyman.com/project/how-to-make-home made-cleaner-with-simple-ingredients

Harvard Health Publishing. (2006, April). *Inflammation: A unifying theory of disease*. Harvard Health. https://www.health.harvard.edu/newsletter_article/Inflammation_A_unifying_theory_of_disease

Harvard Health Publishing. (2018, November 7). *Foods that fight inflammation*. Harvard Health. https://www.health.harvard.edu/staying-healthy/foods-that-fight-inflammation

Harvard Health Publishing. (2020, July 6). *Understanding the stress response*. Harvard Health. https://www.health.harvard.edu/staying-healthy/understanding-the-stress-response

Hill, A. (2019, November 21). *10 interesting types of magnesium*. Healthline. https://www.healthline.com/nutrition/magnesium-types

Hopkinson, E. P. (2022, May 5). *Are your female hormones sabotaging your weight loss?* Medichecks. https://www.medichecks.com/blogs/news/are-your-female-hormones-sabotaging-your-weight-loss

Huizen, J. (2023, January 11). *Hormonal imbalance: Symptoms, causes, and treatment.* https://www.medicalnewstoday.com/articles/321486

Ishler, J. (2021, September 16). *Are you carrying "emotional baggage" here's how to break free.* Healthline. https://www.healthline.com/health/mind-body/how-to-release-emotional-baggage-and-the-tension-that-goes-with-it

Jeffery, S. (2014, June 4). *7 steps to discovering your personal core values.* https://scottjeffrey.com/personal-core-values/

Kearns, A. (2017). *Adrenal fatigue: What causes it?* Mayo Clinic. https://www.mayoclinic.org/diseases-conditions/addisons-disease/expert-answers/adrenal-fatigue/faq-20057906

Kent, G. (2022, May 17). *Motivational quotes for when you need a positive mindset shift.* Www.angelabrown.org. https://www.angelabrown.org/motivational-quotes-for-when-you-need-a-positive-mindset-shift

Khalesi, Z. B., Beiranvand, S. P., & Bokaie, M. (2019). Efficacy of chamomile in the treatment of premenstrual syndrome: A systematic review. *Journal of Pharmacopuncture, 22*(4), 204–209. https://doi.org/10.3831/KPI.2019.22.028

Khatri, S. (2018, April 14). *Hormonal imbalance in women over fifty.* Steady Health. https://www.steadyhealth.com/articles/hormonal-imbalance-in-women-over-fifty

Lawler, M. (2019, October 7). *Beginner's guide to a plant-based diet: Food list, meal plan, benefits, and more.* Everyday Health. https://www.everydayhealth.com/diet-nutrition/plant-based-diet-food-list-meal-plan-benefits-more/

Lidicker, G. (2022, October 7). *Hormonal imbalance treatment: The most common imbalances and what you can do.* Parsley Health. https://www.parsleyhealth.com/blog/what-is-hormonal-imbalance-treatment/

Marcin, A. (2018, August 28). *Emotional eating: What you should know.* Healthline; Healthline Media. https://www.healthline.com/health/emotional-eating

Mariette. (n.d.). *Recipes for the menopause and beyond.* Women's Health Concern. https://www.womens-health-concern.org/help-and-advice/healthy-menopause/recipes/

Mariong Luck Clinic. (2021, September 6). *How does food affect your hormones?.* Mariong Gluck Clinic. https://www.mariongluckclinic.com/blog/how-does-food-affect-your-hormones.html

Mawer, R. (2020, October 22). *The ketogenic diet: A detailed beginner's guide to keto.* Healthline. https://www.healthline.com/nutrition/ketogenic-diet-101

Mayo Clinic. (n.d.). *Free blood pressure machines: Are they accurate?* Mayo Clinic. Retrieved April, 2023, from https://www.mayoclinic.org/diseases-conditions/menopause/expert-answers/hormone-imbalance/faq-20058474

McDonough, L. S. (2020, March 13). *How to DIY an all-purpose cleaner that actually works.* Good Housekeeping. https://www.goodhousekeeping.com/home/cleaning/tips/a24885/make-at-home-cleaners/

McEwen, B. S. (1999). *Endocrine effects on the brain and their relationship to behavior.* Basic Neurochemistry: Molecular, Cellular and Medical Aspects. 6th Edition. https://www.ncbi.nlm.nih.gov/books/NBK20431/

McRae, L. (2019, September 25). *How to start a new routine and stick to it.* Northshore. https://www.northshore.org/healthy-you/how-to-start-a-new-routine-and-stick-to-it/

Mehmet Oz. (n.d.). *Mehmet oz quotes.* BrainyQuote. Retrieved April, 2023, from https://www.brainyquote.com/quotes/mehmet_oz_433794

Miller, R. (2022, April 9). *Keto & menopause: Low-carb diet can "balance hormones" for weight loss.* Express. https://www.express.co.uk/life-style/diets/1592318/Keto-diet-low-carb-menopause-balance-hormones-weight-loss-exclusive

Mindful. (2019, April 13). *How to meditate.* Mindful. https://www.mindful.org/how-to-meditate/

Mumusoglu, S., & Yildiz, B. O. (2020). Polycystic ovary syndrome phenotypes and prevalence: Differential impact of diagnostic criteria and clinical versus unselected population. *Current Opinion in Endocrine and Metabolic Research, 12*, 66–71. https://doi.org/10. 1016/j.coemr.2020.03.004

National Institute of Diabetes and Digestive and Kidney Diseases. (2019, November 19). *Weight management.* National Institute of Diabetes and Digestive and Kidney Diseases. https://www.niddk. nih.gov/health-information/weight-management

National Institute of Environmental Health Sciences. (2018a). *Bisphenol A (BPA).* National Institute of Environmental Health Sciences. https://www.niehs.nih.gov/health/topics/agents/sya-bpa/ index.cfm

National Institute of Environmental Health Sciences. (2018b). *Endocrine disruptors.* National Institute of Environmental Health Sciences. https://www.niehs.nih.gov/health/topics/agents/ endocrine/index.cfm

National Institute of Mental Health. (2019, February 6). *Depression.* National Institute of Mental Health. https://www.nimh.nih.gov/ health/topics/depression/index.shtml

National Institute of Mental Health. (2021). *Caring for your mental health.* Www.nimh.nih.gov. https://www.nimh.nih.gov/health/ topics/caring-for-your-mental-health

National Library Of Medicine. (2020, July 2). *Menopause: What are the benefits and risks of long-term hormone therapy?* Institute for Quality and Efficiency in Health Care (IQWiG). https://www.ncbi.nlm.nih. gov/books/NBK564986/

Nelson, J. (2021, May 12). *Certain foods can aggravate changes during menopause.* The Checkup. https://www.singlecare.com/blog/ menopause-diet/

NHS . (2022, May 17). *Menopause.* NHS. https://www.nhs.uk/condi tions/menopause/

NHS. (2019). *Symptoms - polycystic ovary syndrome.* NHS. https://www. nhs.uk/conditions/polycystic-ovary-syndrome-pcos/symptoms/

NHS. (2021, February 2). *Breathing exercises for stress.* NHS. https:// www.nhs.uk/mental-health/self-help/guides-tools-and-activities/ breathing-exercises-for-stress/

NHS. (2022, September 26). *Reframing unhelpful thoughts - self-help CBT techniques*. NHS. https://www.nhs.uk/every-mind-matters/mental-wellbeing-tips/self-help-cbt-techniques/reframing-unhelpful-thoughts/

NMD, S. S. (2022, July 31). *Best supplements and vitamins to balance hormones*. Women's Health Network. https://www.womenshealth network.com/hormonal-imbalance/best-supplements-and-vita mins-to-balance-hormones/

November 27th, & 2018. (2018, November 27). *11 unexpected signs of hormonal imbalance* Northwell https://www.northwell.edu/obstet rics-and-gynecology/fertility/expert-insights/11-unexpected-signs-of-hormonal-imbalance

OASH. (2019, January 30). *Endometriosis*. Womenshealth.gov. https://www.womenshealth.gov/a-z-topics/endometriosis

Ostermeyer, K. (2021, January 3). *Pros and cons of alternative medicine, modern medicine and traditional medicine*. Elite Learning. https://www.elitelearning.com/resource-center/nursing/pros-cons-of-alternative-medicine-modern-medicine-traditional-medicine/

Pacheco, D. (2021, January 8). *How to build a better bedtime routine for adults*. Sleep Foundation. https://www.sleepfoundation.org/sleep-hygiene/bedtime-routine-for-adults

Paracelsus. (n.d.). *Paracelsus quotes*. BrainyQuote. https://www.brainyquote.com/quotes/paracelsus_170321

Parsley Health. (2016, July 16). *Hormonal imbalance symptoms & treatment: 10 ways to balance them naturally*. Parsley Health. https://www.parsleyhealth.com/blog/hormonal-imbalance-symptoms/

Peters, B. (2019). *How to ruin sleep: 10 bad habits and the worst ways to cause insomnia*. Verywell Health. https://www.verywellhealth.com/the-10-worst-ways-to-ruin-your-sleep-3014992

Pick, M., OB/GYN, & NP. (2018, August 5). *7 essential oils for hormones*. Marcelle Pick, OB/GYN NP. https://marcellepick.com/7-essential-oils-for-hormones/

Postmenopause: Signs, symptoms & what to expect. (2021, May 10). Cleveland Clinic. https://my.clevelandclinic.org/health/diseases/21837-postmenopause

Publishing, H. H. (2023, April 15). *Quick-start guide to an anti-inflamma-tion diet*. Harvard Health. https://www.health.harvard.edu/staying-healthy/quick-start-guide-to-an-antiinflammation-diet

Reinagel, N. D. M. (2016, November 23). *How does dairy affect your hormone levels?* Scientific American. https://www.scientificameri can.com/article/how-does-dairy-affect-your-hormone-levels

Reynolds, G. (2021, September 29). *Why exercise is more important than weight loss for a longer life*. The New York Times. https://www.nytimes.com/2021/09/29/well/move/exercise-weight-loss-longer-life.html#:

Roland, J. (2023, March 9). *Signs of insulin resistance*. Healthline. https://www.healthline.com/health/diabetes/insulin-resistance-symptoms

Rose, A. (2021, July 22). *How female hormones affect exercise — at every age*. Healthline. https://www.healthline.com/health/fitness/how-female-hormones-affect-exercise-at-every-age

Rowles, A. (2017, April 10). *12 simple tips to prevent blood sugar spikes*. Healthline; Healthline Media. https://www.healthline.com/nutri tion/blood-sugar-spikes

Schopenhauer, A. (n.d.). *Arthur Schopenhauer quotes*. BrainyQuote. Retrieved April 28, 2023, from https://www.brainyquote.com/quotes/arthur_schopenhauer_103608?src=t_truth

Shomon , M. (2022, December 23). *What to know about selenium and your thyroid*. Verywell Health. https://www.verywellhealth.com/sele nium-and-your-thyroid-4134998

Silva, A. M. C., Campos, P. H. N., Mattos, I. E., Hajat, S., Lacerda, E. M., & Ferreira, M. J. M. (2019). Environmental exposure to pesticides and breast cancer in a region of intensive agribusiness activity in brazil: A case-control study. *International Journal of Environmental Research and Public Health, 16*(20), 3951. https://doi.org/10.3390/ijerph16203951

Sweetser, R. (2022, May 5). *5 homemade pesticides: Soap sprays for plants*. Almanac.com. https://www.almanac.com/organic-pesticides

Synder, C. (2021, June 23). *5 impressive herbs that help balance your hormones*. Healthline. https://www.healthline.com/nutrition/herbs-that-balance-hormones

Teede, H. J., & Boyle, J. (2012). *Polycystic ovary syndrome*. Australian Family Physician. https://www.racgp.org.au/afp/2012/october/ polycystic-ovary-syndrome

Tennant, L. (2021, February 19). *Iodine & thyroid health: Are you getting enough?* | imaware™. Www.imaware.health. https://www.imaware. health/blog/iodine-and-thyroid-health

UK, A. (2021, November 22). *10 homemade beauty products you need to try*. Aromantic UK. https://aromantic.co.uk/blogs/aromantic-blog/ 10-homemade-beauty-products-to-try

WebMD. (2002, October 7). *Menopause basics*. WebMD. https://www. webmd.com/menopause/guide/menopause-basics

WebMD. (2023). *Food & recipes*. WebMD. https://www.webmd.com/ food-recipes/features/10-tips-for-healthy-grocery-shopping#:

World Health Organization. (2023, March 24). *Endometriosis*. World Health Organization. https://www.who.int/news-room/fact-sheets/detail/endometriosis

Yates, A. (2022, July 7). *7 apps to help you monitor and understand your hormonal balance*. MUO. https://www.makeuseof.com/apps-moni tor-understand-hormonal-balance/

Yetman, D. (2020, November 25). *How to go back to sleep after waking up at night: 10 tips, prevention*. Healthline. https://www.healthline.com/ health/how-to-go-back-to-sleep

Young, S. H. (2007, August 14). *18 tricks to make new habits stick*. Lifehack. https://www.lifehack.org/articles/featured/18-tricks-to-make-new-habits-stick.html

Zizinia, S. (2022, April 26). *5 common myths about hormone imbalances*. MD Anderson Cancer Center. https://www.mdanderson.org/ cancerwise/5-common-myths-about-hormone-imbalances-and-thyroid-function.h00-159538956.html

Printed in Great Britain
by Amazon

29734312R00117